PRAISES

"Evelyn Green has cracked the code to sustainable weight loss! This book is a game-changer, offering a holistic approach that nourishes the body and mind. The 28-day plan is easy to follow, the recipes are delicious, and the insights into green tea's benefits are truly enlightening. I've lost weight, gained energy, and feel more empowered than ever before!" - Sarah M.

"I've tried countless diets and workout plans, but nothing has worked as well as the Green Tea Metabolism Makeover. This book has taught me how to make sustainable lifestyle changes that have transformed my relationship with food and exercise. I'm not just losing weight; I'm gaining a healthier, happier life!" –

David L.

"As a green tea enthusiast, I was thrilled to discover this book. It's a treasure trove of information on green tea's amazing benefits, from boosting metabolism to promoting gut health and reducing stress. The recipes are creative and delicious, and the 28-day plan is a fantastic way to incorporate green tea into your daily routine. I highly recommend this book to anyone seeking a natural and sustainable path to wellness." - Emily R.

"Evelyn Green's writing style is engaging and informative, making complex concepts easy to understand. I appreciate the holistic approach to weight loss, which addresses not only diet and exercise but also stress management and sleep. The Green Tea Metabolism Makeover is a must-read for anyone looking to transform their health and well-being from the inside out." - Michael T.

"This book is a breath of fresh air in the often overwhelming world of weight loss. Evelyn Green's passion for green tea and her commitment to sustainable health shine through on every page. The Green Tea Metabolism Makeover is a practical, informative, and inspiring guide that has empowered me to make lasting changes and embrace a more vibrant life. Thank you, Evelyn!" - Jessica K.

THE GREEN TEA METABOLISM MAKEOVER

A 28-Day Plan to Ignite Your Fat-Burning Engine, Revitalize Your Energy, and Shed Pounds Naturally

Evelyn Green

Table of content

Acknowledgments

This book wouldn't have been possible without the support and encouragement of many individuals.

First and foremost, I extend my deepest gratitude to my family and friends, who patiently listened to my endless ramblings about green tea and metabolism. Your love and unwavering belief in me fueled my passion and kept me motivated throughout the writing process.

I'm also grateful to the countless researchers and scientists who have dedicated their careers to unraveling the mysteries of green tea and its impact on human health. Your tireless efforts have provided the scientific foundation upon which this book is built.

To the tea farmers and producers around the world, thank you for cultivating and crafting this remarkable beverage that has brought joy and well-being to countless individuals throughout history.

And finally, to you, the reader, thank you for embarking on this journey with me. I hope that this book inspires and empowers you to embrace the power of green tea and create a healthier, happier life.

May your cup always be full of warmth, flavor, and good health.

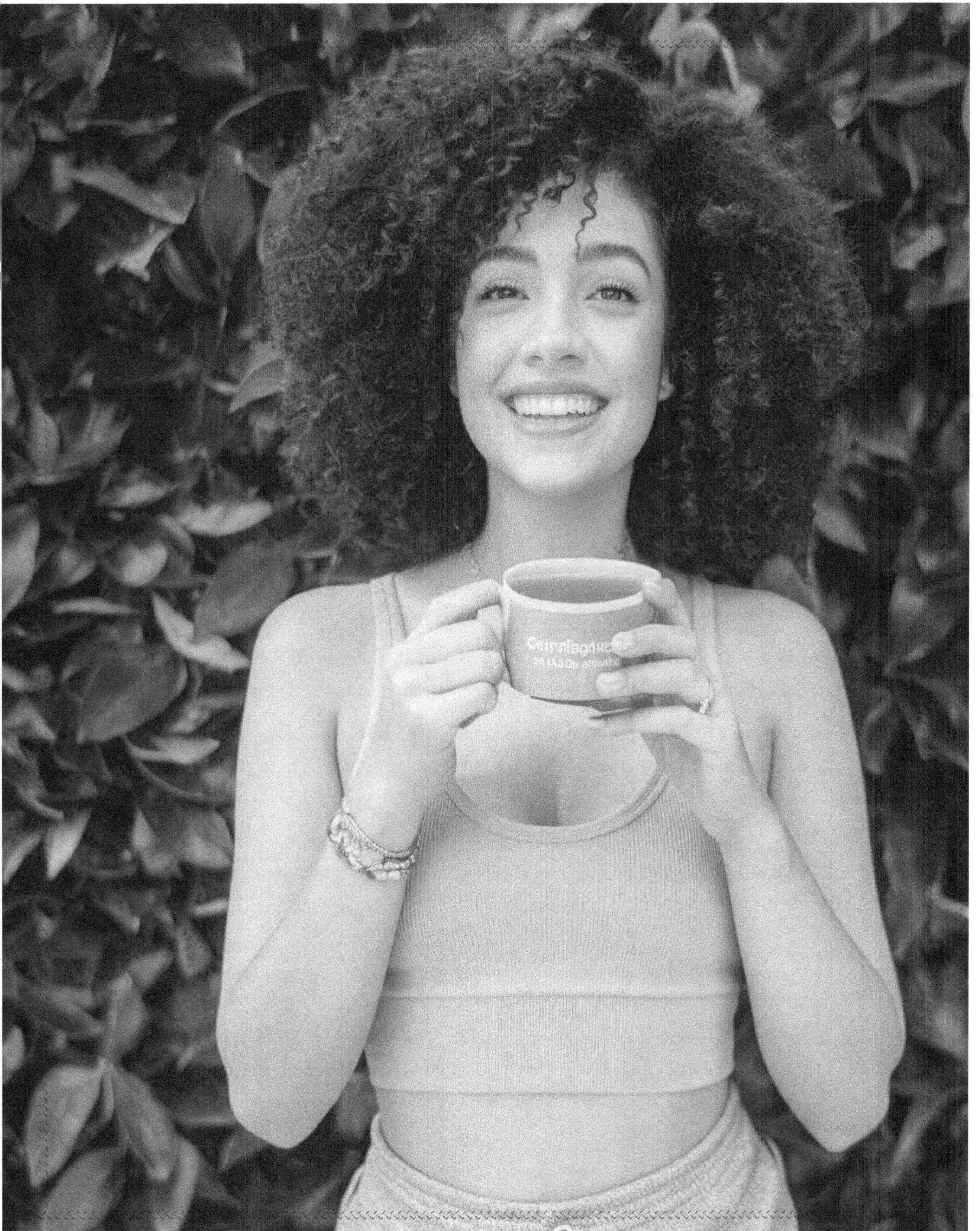

INTRODUCTION

"Nature itself is the best physician." – Hippocrates

The mirror wasn't my friend. Every glance felt like a confrontation, a stark reminder of the extra pounds that clung stubbornly to my frame. I was trapped in a cycle of fad diets and yo-yo weight loss, my energy levels perpetually low, and my self-esteem taking a nosedive. I yearned for a solution that wasn't just about shedding weight but about revitalizing my entire being.

Then, during a trip to Japan, I stumbled upon a centuries-old tradition that would change my life: the Japanese tea ceremony. As I watched the tea master meticulously prepare matcha, a vibrant green tea powder, I was struck by the reverence and intentionality surrounding this simple act. It wasn't just about drinking tea; it was about mindfulness, connection, and nourishment.

Intrigued, I took my first sip of matcha and experienced an awakening. A gentle wave of energy washed over me, replacing the usual afternoon slump with a sense of calm focus. The earthy flavor was both invigorating and soothing, a welcome contrast to the sugary drinks I had relied on for so long.

Little did I know that this unassuming cup of green tea was about to ignite a transformation that would ripple through every aspect of my life.

The Ancient Elixir, Backed by Modern Science

Green tea, revered for centuries in various cultures for its medicinal properties, is far more than just a comforting beverage. It's a treasure trove of antioxidants, vitamins, and minerals, including the potent compound EGCG, renowned for its metabolism-boosting and fat-burning capabilities.

Modern science has confirmed what ancient wisdom has long known: green tea is a powerful ally in the quest for a healthier, leaner body. Studies have shown that it can increase metabolism, enhance fat oxidation, and even help regulate appetite. But its benefits extend far beyond weight loss, offering a holistic approach to well-being that nourishes your body and mind from the inside out.

"The Green Tea Metabolism Makeover" isn't just another diet book. It's your personal invitation to a 28-day journey of transformation, guided by the wisdom of ancient traditions and the power of modern science. It's about creating a sustainable lifestyle that not only helps you shed unwanted pounds but also revitalizes your energy, improves your mood, and empowers you to embrace a healthier, happier you.

In these pages, you'll discover:

The Science of Green Tea: We'll delve into the fascinating world of green tea's unique compounds, unraveling the mechanisms behind its metabolism-boosting and fat-burning effects. You'll gain a deeper understanding of how this ancient elixir can support your weight loss goals and enhance your overall health.

The 28-Day Plan: We'll guide you through a transformative 28-day journey, seamlessly integrating green tea into your daily routine. From invigorating matcha lattes to refreshing iced teas and even creative culinary uses, you'll discover a world of flavors and possibilities that make green tea an enjoyable and sustainable part of your lifestyle.

The Green Tea Metabolism Meal Plan: Say goodbye to restrictive diets and hello to a balanced and nourishing meal plan that complements the effects of green tea. We'll focus on whole, nutrient-dense foods that fuel your metabolism, promote satiety, and support your weight loss goals. You'll also find a collection of mouthwatering recipes that incorporate green tea, adding an extra boost of flavor and antioxidants to your meals.

The Green Tea Workout: Ignite your fat-burning potential with a tailored exercise plan that combines cardio and strength training. We'll guide you through effective workouts that complement your green tea-powered lifestyle, helping you achieve your fitness goals and enhance your overall well-being.

Mind, Body, and Green Tea: We'll explore the intricate connection between stress, sleep, and gut health with weight management. Discover how green tea can promote relaxation, improve sleep quality, and support a healthy gut microbiome, all of which play crucial roles in achieving and maintaining a healthy weight.

Beyond Weight Loss: Uncover the myriad of additional health benefits that green tea offers, from heart health to cognitive function and radiant skin. You'll learn how this versatile beverage can enhance your overall well-being and protect against chronic diseases, empowering you to live a longer, healthier, and more fulfilling life.

Just like my own transformative experience with green tea, I believe that this book has the power to inspire and empower you to embark on your own journey toward a healthier, happier you. It's not about perfection or deprivation; it's about progress, self-discovery, and embracing a lifestyle that nourishes your body and mind.

Let's turn the page together and begin your Green Tea Metabolism Makeover. With each step, you'll uncover the hidden potential within you, igniting your metabolism, revitalizing your energy, and radiating confidence from the inside out. Your transformation awaits.

Chapter 1: The Green Elixir: Unveiling the Magic of Green Tea

"Better to be deprived of food for three days, than tea for one." – Ancient Chinese Proverb

The world of weight loss is often shrouded in mystery, misinformation, and fleeting trends. We're constantly bombarded with promises of rapid results from dubious supplements and extreme diets. Yet, amidst this chaos, there exists a humble, time-tested elixir that has quietly revolutionized the way we approach health and well-being. It's a beverage steeped in history, brimming with scientific validation, and celebrated for its remarkable ability to ignite our metabolism and unlock our body's fat-burning potential.

Welcome to the enchanting world of green tea, the star of our "Green Tea Metabolism Makeover."

1.1. A Brief History of Green Tea: From Ancient Ritual to Modern Health Phenomenon

Our journey begins in ancient China, where green tea first emerged as a revered beverage over 4,000 years ago. Legend has it that Emperor Shennong, a scholar and herbalist, discovered the invigorating properties of tea when leaves from a Camellia sinensis plant accidentally fell into his boiling water. Intrigued by the resulting brew's aroma and taste, he took a sip and was instantly captivated by its revitalizing effects.

From that serendipitous moment, green tea became an integral part of Chinese culture, valued for its medicinal properties and used in traditional ceremonies and rituals.

Buddhist monks, renowned for their disciplined lifestyle and pursuit of enlightenment, adopted green tea as a means to enhance focus and concentration during meditation.

Over centuries, green tea's popularity spread throughout Asia, reaching Japan, where it evolved into an art form. The Japanese tea ceremony, known as Chanoyu or Sado, is a meticulously choreographed ritual that celebrates the preparation and consumption of matcha, a finely ground green tea powder. Matcha's vibrant green color and unique umami flavor have made it a sought-after ingredient in both traditional and modern culinary creations.

In the 17th century, green tea made its way to Europe through Dutch traders, captivating the continent with its exotic allure and purported health benefits. It soon became a fashionable beverage among the aristocracy, enjoyed in elegant tea salons and porcelain cups.

Today, green tea's popularity has reached unprecedented heights, transcending cultural boundaries and becoming a global phenomenon. Its reputation as a health-promoting beverage is supported by a wealth of scientific research, revealing its potential to aid in weight loss, improve heart health, boost brain function, and even protect against certain types of cancer.

1.2. The Science Behind the Brew: Green Tea's Unique Compounds and Their Health Benefits

What makes green tea such a potent elixir for health and weight loss? The answer lies in its unique composition of bioactive compounds, each playing a crucial role in promoting our well-being.

- **Catechins:** These powerful antioxidants are the most abundant and well-studied components of green tea. They possess remarkable anti-inflammatory, anti-cancer, and anti-obesity properties. The most potent catechin, epigallocatechin gallate (EGCG), has been extensively researched for its ability to boost metabolism, increase fat oxidation, and reduce fat cell development.

- **L-theanine:** This amino acid, found almost exclusively in tea plants, is responsible for green tea's calming and relaxing effects. It counteracts the jittery side effects of caffeine, promoting a state of focused alertness and tranquility. L-theanine also enhances cognitive function, memory, and mood.

- **Caffeine:** While present in lower amounts than coffee, green tea still contains a moderate amount of caffeine, providing a gentle energy boost and increased alertness. Caffeine has also been shown to enhance athletic performance and increase fat burning during exercise.
- **Other Bioactive Compounds:** Green tea also contains a variety of other beneficial compounds, including vitamins, minerals, and flavonoids, which contribute to its overall health-promoting effects.

The synergistic action of these compounds makes green tea a true powerhouse for weight loss and metabolic enhancement. Studies have shown that regular consumption of green tea can:

- **Increase metabolism:** Green tea's catechins and caffeine work together to boost thermogenesis, the process of heat production in the body that burns calories. This can lead to an increase in daily energy expenditure, helping you burn more calories even at rest.
- **Enhance fat oxidation:** EGCG, the most potent catechin in green tea, has been shown to increase fat oxidation, the process of breaking down stored fat for energy. This can help you reduce body fat and achieve a leaner physique.
- **Suppress appetite:** Green tea may help curb appetite and reduce cravings, potentially leading to lower calorie intake and weight loss.
- **Improve insulin sensitivity:** Some research suggests that green tea may help improve insulin sensitivity, making it easier for your body to use glucose for energy and reducing the risk of insulin resistance, a precursor to type 2 diabetes.

In addition to its weight loss benefits, green tea has been associated with a wide range of other health advantages, including:

-

- **Improved heart health:** Green tea may help lower LDL ("bad") cholesterol and triglyceride levels, while increasing HDL ("good") cholesterol. It may also help reduce blood pressure and improve blood vessel function.

- **Enhanced brain function:** The combination of caffeine and L-theanine in green tea has been shown to improve cognitive function, memory, attention, and reaction time. Green tea may also have neuroprotective effects, potentially reducing the risk of neurodegenerative diseases like Alzheimer's and Parkinson's.
- **Reduced risk of cancer:** Studies suggest that the antioxidants in green tea may help protect against various types of cancer, including breast, colon, prostate, and lung cancer.
- **Healthier skin:** Green tea's antioxidants can protect the skin from damage caused by free radicals, which are unstable molecules that can accelerate aging and contribute to wrinkles and fine lines. Green tea may also help reduce inflammation and improve skin elasticity.

As we embark on this transformative journey together, we'll delve deeper into the science behind green tea, exploring the mechanisms through which it works its magic on our metabolism and overall health. We'll uncover the different types of green tea, learn how to brew the perfect cup, and discover creative ways to incorporate it into our daily lives.

Chapter 2: Reving Up Your Metabolism: Green Tea's Fat-Burning Power

In our quest to ignite our metabolism and unlock the fat-burning power of green tea, it's essential to first understand the intricate workings of our body's energy engine: metabolism. Imagine your metabolism as a complex network of biochemical reactions constantly humming within your cells, converting the food you eat into energy that fuels your every move, thought, and bodily function. It's the invisible force that dictates how efficiently you burn calories, utilize nutrients, and maintain your ideal body composition.

At its core, metabolism is a dynamic process composed of two key components: basal metabolic rate (BMR) and total daily energy expenditure (TDEE). Your BMR represents the minimum number of calories your body requires to sustain essential functions at rest. This includes the energy needed for breathing, circulating blood, maintaining body temperature, and powering your organs. Think of it as the energy your body burns simply to keep you alive and functioning, even while you're asleep or relaxing.

However, your body's energy needs extend beyond just resting functions. Total daily energy expenditure (TDEE) encompasses all the calories you burn throughout the day, including those used for physical activity, digestion, and other bodily processes. It's the sum of your BMR, the energy used for physical activity, and the thermic effect of food (TEF), which is the energy required to digest and process the food you eat.

Picture your BMR as the engine idling in your car, while TDEE is the engine revving up during an exhilarating drive. Your BMR accounts for a significant portion of your TDEE, typically ranging from 60% to 75%. This means that even when you're not actively exercising, your body is still burning a considerable amount of calories just to keep you alive.

The remaining 25% to 40% of your TDEE is determined by your activity level, the thermic effect of food, and non-exercise activity thermogenesis (NEAT). NEAT encompasses all the calories burned through everyday movements like fidgeting, standing, walking, and even typing.

Several factors influence your metabolism, making it a unique and ever-changing process for each individual. Age is a significant factor, as metabolism tends to gradually slow down with each passing decade. This is primarily due to a natural decline in muscle mass and hormonal changes associated with aging. Gender also plays a role, with men generally having higher BMRs than women due to their larger body size and greater muscle mass.

Body composition, particularly the ratio of lean muscle mass to fat, significantly impacts your metabolism. Muscle is a metabolically active tissue, meaning it burns more calories even at rest compared to fat. Therefore, increasing muscle mass through strength training can be an effective way to boost your metabolism and enhance fat burning. Genetics also play a crucial role in determining your metabolic rate. Some individuals are naturally predisposed to having a faster or slower metabolism due to genetic variations. However, it's important to note that while genetics provide a blueprint, your lifestyle choices can significantly influence how your genes express themselves. Through regular exercise, a balanced diet rich in whole foods, adequate sleep, and stress management, you can optimize your metabolism and take control of your weight loss journey.

This is where green tea enters the picture as a powerful ally. Green tea's unique blend of bioactive compounds, particularly catechins like EGCG, has been shown to directly influence several aspects of metabolism, making it a valuable tool for weight management. Research suggests that green tea can increase thermogenesis, the process of heat production in the body that burns calories. By activating specific enzymes and pathways, green tea can give your BMR a boost, helping you burn more calories even while you're relaxing. This effect is further enhanced when combined with the caffeine naturally present in green tea, which has been shown to increase energy expenditure and fat oxidation.

Furthermore, green tea's ability to enhance fat oxidation means that your body becomes more efficient at using stored fat for energy. This not only contributes to weight loss but also improves your body composition by reducing fat mass and potentially increasing lean muscle mass, which further boosts your metabolism.

In addition to its direct effects on BMR and fat oxidation, green tea may also influence other aspects of your metabolism. For instance, some studies suggest that green tea can improve insulin sensitivity, making it easier for your body to utilize glucose for energy and reducing the risk of insulin resistance, a major contributor to metabolic syndrome and type 2 diabetes.

By incorporating green tea into your daily routine, adopting a balanced meal plan, and engaging in regular exercise, you can create a synergistic effect that optimizes your metabolism and unlocks your body's fat-burning potential. The 28-day Green Tea Metabolism Makeover plan provides a comprehensive roadmap to guide you through this transformative journey, empowering you to achieve sustainable weight loss and optimal health.

Green Tea and Thermogenesis: Turning Up the Heat on Fat Burning

Imagine your body as a furnace, constantly generating heat to keep you warm and energized. This internal heat production, known as thermogenesis, is a crucial component of your metabolism and plays a significant role in how efficiently you burn calories and manage your weight. In essence, thermogenesis is the process by which your body converts stored energy (calories) into heat, a byproduct of various metabolic processes.

Think of it this way: every time you eat, your body expends energy to digest, absorb, and metabolize the nutrients from your food. This process, called the thermic effect of food (TEF), contributes to thermogenesis. Additionally, physical activity, whether it's a brisk walk or an intense workout, generates heat as your muscles contract and burn calories for fuel. Even shivering when you're cold is a form of thermogenesis, as your body attempts to raise its temperature.

Thermogenesis isn't just about staying warm; it's a key player in weight management. The more heat your body produces, the more calories you burn, creating a calorie deficit that can lead to weight loss. This is where green tea enters the picture, wielding its thermogenic power to amplify your body's fat-burning capabilities.

Green tea's secret weapon lies in its unique combination of catechins, particularly epigallocatechin gallate (EGCG), and caffeine. These compounds work synergistically to ignite your internal furnace, increasing thermogenesis and boosting your metabolic rate. EGCG, the most abundant and potent catechin in green tea, has been extensively studied for its thermogenic properties. Research suggests that EGCG can stimulate brown adipose tissue (BAT), a type of fat that specializes in generating heat. Unlike white adipose tissue (WAT), which stores energy, BAT burns calories to produce heat, contributing to thermogenesis.

EGCG activates BAT by increasing the levels of norepinephrine, a hormone that triggers fat breakdown and heat production. Additionally, EGCG has been shown to inhibit an enzyme called catechol-O-methyltransferase (COMT), which breaks down norepinephrine. By inhibiting COMT, EGCG prolongs the action of norepinephrine, further enhancing thermogenesis.

Caffeine, another key component of green tea, also plays a role in boosting thermogenesis. It stimulates the central nervous system, increasing heart rate and metabolic rate. This leads to a higher calorie burn, even at rest. Furthermore, caffeine works synergistically with EGCG, enhancing its thermogenic effects. Studies have shown that the combination of EGCG and caffeine can increase energy expenditure by up to 10%, translating to an extra 100-200 calories burned per day.

The impact of green tea on thermogenesis isn't limited to just a few hours after consumption. Research suggests that regular intake of green tea can lead to sustained increases in thermogenesis over time, helping you maintain a higher metabolic rate and burn more calories in the long run.

Incorporating green tea into your daily routine is a simple yet effective way to turn up the heat on your fat-burning engine. Whether you prefer it hot or iced, brewed from loose leaves or enjoyed as a matcha latte, green tea offers a delicious and refreshing way to boost your metabolism and support your weight loss goals. Aim to consume 2-3 cups of green tea per day to maximize its thermogenic benefits.

But remember, green tea isn't a magic bullet. While it can significantly enhance thermogenesis, it's most effective when combined with a healthy diet and regular exercise. The 28-Day Green Tea Metabolism Makeover plan provides a comprehensive approach to weight loss, incorporating green tea alongside a balanced meal plan and exercise routine to optimize your results. By adopting this holistic approach, you'll create a sustainable lifestyle that not only promotes weight loss but also enhances your overall health and well-being.

The Role of Catechins: Green Tea's Metabolic Superstars

Within the emerald depths of green tea lies a treasure trove of compounds known as catechins, the unsung heroes of metabolism and fat burning. These naturally occurring antioxidants are the key to unlocking green tea's transformative power, working tirelessly behind the scenes to rev up your metabolic engine and help you achieve your weight loss goals.

Among the catechins, one stands out as the undisputed champion: epigallocatechin gallate, or EGCG for short. This remarkable compound has captured the attention of scientists and health enthusiasts alike due to its exceptional ability to promote fat oxidation, inhibit fat storage, and enhance overall metabolic function. In essence, EGCG acts as a metabolic catalyst, accelerating the processes that convert stored fat into usable energy.

How does EGCG work its magic? It all starts with fat oxidation, the process by which your body breaks down fat molecules to release energy. EGCG has been shown to increase the activity of enzymes involved in fat oxidation, essentially turning up the dial on your body's fat-burning furnace. This leads to a greater utilization of stored fat for energy, contributing to weight loss and a leaner physique.

But EGCG doesn't stop there. It also inhibits the activity of enzymes that promote fat storage, making it harder for your body to accumulate new fat deposits. This dual action of increasing fat burning and reducing fat storage is a powerful combination for achieving sustainable weight loss. Numerous scientific studies have validated the metabolic benefits of EGCG. A landmark study published in the American Journal of Clinical Nutrition found that green tea extract containing EGCG significantly increased 24-hour energy expenditure and fat oxidation compared to a placebo. Another study in the Journal of Nutrition demonstrated that EGCG supplementation led to a reduction in body fat and waist circumference in overweight and obese individuals.

EGCG's effects extend beyond fat metabolism. Research suggests that it may also enhance insulin sensitivity, the ability of your body to respond to insulin and regulate blood sugar levels. Improved insulin sensitivity is crucial for weight management, as it helps prevent the storage of excess glucose as fat. Furthermore, EGCG has been shown to increase the levels of norepinephrine, a hormone that plays a key role in fat breakdown. By boosting norepinephrine, EGCG further enhances your body's ability to mobilize and utilize stored fat for energy.

The combined effects of EGCG on fat oxidation, fat storage, insulin sensitivity, and norepinephrine make it a true metabolic superstar. And the best part is that you don't need to isolate EGCG to reap its benefits; simply enjoying a few cups of green tea each day can provide you with a significant dose of this potent compound. The 28-day Green Tea Metabolism Makeover plan strategically incorporates green tea into your daily routine to maximize your exposure to EGCG and other beneficial catechins. By sipping on green tea throughout the day, you'll be fueling your body with a natural and effective fat-burning elixir.

Remember, the journey to a healthier, leaner you is not about quick fixes or fad diets. It's about making sustainable lifestyle changes that support your body's natural processes. Green tea, with its remarkable array of catechins, including the mighty EGCG, is a powerful tool that can help you achieve your goals and transform your metabolism. As you embark on this makeover, embrace the power of green tea and allow its catechins to work their magic, igniting your fat-burning potential and paving the way for a healthier, more vibrant you. With each sip, you're not just enjoying a delicious beverage; you're investing in your metabolic health and unlocking the secrets to sustainable weight loss.

Chapter 3: The 28-Day Green Tea Metabolism Makeover: Your Roadmap to Success

Embarking on a transformative journey towards a healthier, leaner you requires more than just good intentions; it demands a well-structured plan that acts as your compass, guiding you through the twists and turns of your weight loss adventure. Think of this plan as your personal roadmap to success, meticulously crafted to optimize your metabolism, nourish your body, and empower you to make lasting changes.

The 28-day Green Tea Metabolism Makeover is not just a random assortment of tips and tricks; it's a carefully designed program that leverages the power of green tea and combines it with a holistic approach to nutrition, exercise, and lifestyle modifications. This structured plan provides you with a clear direction, ensuring that you stay focused, motivated, and on track to achieve your goals.

Why is a structured plan so crucial for weight loss? Research has consistently shown that individuals who follow a well-defined plan are more likely to succeed in their weight loss endeavors compared to those who take a haphazard approach. A plan eliminates guesswork, reduces decision fatigue, and provides a sense of accountability, making it easier to stick to your healthy habits even when faced with challenges or temptations.

The 28-day Green Tea Metabolism Makeover is your comprehensive blueprint for success. It encompasses four key components that work synergistically to transform your body and mind:

1. **Daily Green Tea Rituals:** Green tea, the cornerstone of this makeover, will become your trusted companion throughout the 28 days. You'll learn to incorporate various types of green tea into your daily routine, savoring its rich flavor and reaping its metabolic benefits. From matcha lattes to invigorating iced teas, you'll discover a plethora of delicious and creative ways to enjoy this elixir. We'll guide you on optimal brewing techniques, ideal consumption times, and the different green tea varieties that best suit your preferences and goals.

2. **The Green Tea Metabolism Meal Plan:** A balanced and nourishing diet is essential for fueling your body, supporting your metabolism, and achieving sustainable weight loss. Our meticulously crafted meal plan is designed to complement the effects of green tea, providing you with the right balance of macronutrients and micronutrients to optimize your health and energy

levels. We'll introduce you to a variety of delicious and satisfying recipes that incorporate green tea, ensuring that your meals are both nutritious and enjoyable. You'll learn to prioritize whole, unprocessed foods, control portion sizes, and make mindful choices that support your weight loss journey.

3. The Green Tea Workout: Exercise is a key component of any successful weight loss plan, and the Green Tea Metabolism Makeover is no exception. We'll provide you with a tailored workout plan that combines cardiovascular exercise for calorie burning with strength training for muscle building and metabolic enhancement. Our workouts are designed to be adaptable to different fitness levels, ensuring that you can participate and progress at your own pace. By incorporating exercise into your daily routine, you'll accelerate your metabolism, build lean muscle mass, and enhance your overall well-being.

4. Lifestyle Modifications: Beyond diet and exercise, certain lifestyle modifications can significantly impact your weight loss journey. We'll explore strategies for managing stress, improving sleep quality, and cultivating a positive mindset, all of which play crucial roles in achieving and maintaining a healthy weight. You'll learn to identify and overcome potential obstacles, develop healthy coping mechanisms, and create a supportive environment for your transformation.

Throughout the 28 days, you'll be encouraged to track your progress, celebrate your achievements, and adjust your plan as needed. Our comprehensive tracking tools will help you monitor your weight, measurements, body composition, energy levels, and overall well-being. This data will provide valuable insights into your progress and empower you to make informed decisions about your health.

Remember, the Green Tea Metabolism Makeover is not a one-size-fits-all solution. It's a personalized journey that caters to your unique needs and preferences. We encourage you to embrace the flexibility of the plan and adapt it to fit your lifestyle. Whether you're a busy professional, a stay-at-home parent, or a student, you can customize the meal plan, exercise routine, and lifestyle modifications to suit your schedule and individual requirements.

By following the Green Tea Metabolism Makeover plan, you'll not only shed pounds and improve your metabolism but also cultivate a healthier relationship with food, exercise, and your body.

You'll develop sustainable habits that will continue to serve you long after the 28 days are over, setting you on a path toward lifelong health and well-being.

Embrace the power of a plan, and let the Green Tea Metabolism Makeover be your guide to a transformed you. With commitment, consistency, and the support of this comprehensive program, you'll unlock your body's full potential and achieve the lasting results you desire.

Daily Green Tea Rituals: Incorporating Green Tea into Your Routine

Embarking on the Green Tea Metabolism Makeover is not about restriction or deprivation; it's about embracing a delightful and invigorating new way of life. In this chapter, we'll explore how to seamlessly weave green tea into your daily routine, transforming it from a mere beverage into a ritual that nourishes your body, mind, and spirit.

Imagine waking up to the vibrant green hue of a matcha latte, its earthy aroma awakening your senses and preparing you for the day ahead. Matcha, a finely ground green tea powder, is renowned for its high concentration of antioxidants, including the metabolism-boosting EGCG. Its invigorating caffeine content provides a gentle, sustained energy boost without the jitters often associated with coffee.

As you transition into your workday, consider sipping on a cup of sencha, the most popular green tea in Japan. Sencha offers a delicate balance of grassy notes, umami, and a subtle sweetness. Its moderate caffeine content can help maintain your focus and productivity throughout the afternoon slump.

For a mid-morning or afternoon pick-me-up, why not try a refreshing iced green tea? Brew a strong batch of your favorite green tea, let it cool, and pour it over ice. You can add a squeeze of lemon or lime for a zesty twist, or infuse it with fruits like berries or peaches for a naturally sweet and flavorful treat. If you're feeling adventurous, experiment with adding herbs like mint, basil, or even a sprig of rosemary for a unique and invigorating flavor profile.

As the day winds down, consider switching to a calming cup of chamomile green tea. This delightful blend combines the soothing properties of chamomile with the metabolism-boosting benefits of green tea. Chamomile has long been used to promote relaxation and sleep, making it the perfect beverage to unwind with before bed.

To add variety and excitement to your green tea routine, let's explore some creative and delicious recipes that go beyond the traditional cup.

Matcha Latte: Start your day with this vibrant and energizing drink. Simply whisk 1 teaspoon of matcha powder with a small amount of hot water until frothy. Then, add 1 cup of your favorite milk (dairy or non-dairy) and sweeten to taste with honey or maple syrup. You can also experiment with adding a pinch of cinnamon, nutmeg, or ginger for an extra flavor boost.

Green Tea Smoothie: Blend 1 cup of brewed and cooled green tea with a handful of spinach, ½ cup of frozen berries, ½ a banana, and a scoop of protein powder for a nutrient-packed breakfast or snack. You can adjust the ingredients to your liking, adding other fruits, vegetables, or superfoods like chia seeds or flaxseed.

Green Tea Lemonade: This refreshing summer drink is perfect for quenching your thirst and boosting your metabolism. Combine 1 cup of brewed and cooled green tea with ½ cup of freshly squeezed lemon juice, ½ cup of water, and sweeten to taste with honey or agave. Garnish with a sprig of mint or a slice of lemon.

Green Tea Popsicles: These healthy and delicious treats are a fun way to enjoy green tea on a hot day. Simply combine 1 cup of brewed and cooled green tea with ½ cup of your favorite juice (such as orange, pineapple, or mango) and sweeten to taste with honey or agave. Pour the mixture into popsicle molds and freeze until solid.

Green Tea Chia Pudding: This creamy and satisfying dessert is packed with fiber and protein, making it a healthy alternative to sugary treats. Combine 1 cup of brewed and cooled green tea with 2 tablespoons of chia seeds, 1 tablespoon of honey or maple syrup, and a pinch of vanilla extract. Stir well and refrigerate for at least 4 hours or overnight. Top with fresh fruit, nuts, or granola before serving.

Green Tea Energy Bites: These bite-sized snacks are perfect for an on-the-go energy boost. Combine 1 cup of rolled oats, ½ cup of nut butter, ¼ cup of honey or maple syrup, 2 tablespoons of green tea powder (matcha), and a pinch of salt. Mix well and roll into small balls. Refrigerate for at least 30 minutes before serving.

These are just a few ideas to get you started on your green tea journey. Feel free to get creative and experiment with different flavors and combinations to find what works best for you. Remember, the key is to make green tea a pleasurable and sustainable part of your daily routine.

To further enhance the benefits of green tea, here are some additional tips:

Choose high-quality tea: Opt for loose leaf tea whenever possible, as it often offers superior flavor and higher antioxidant content compared to tea bags.

Brew it right: Follow the instructions on your tea package for the ideal water temperature and steeping time. Over-brewing can result in a bitter taste, while under-brewing may not extract all the beneficial compounds.

Drink it throughout the day: Aim to spread your green tea intake throughout the day rather than consuming it all at once. This will help maintain a steady supply of antioxidants and energy-boosting compounds in your system.

Experiment with different varieties: There are numerous types of green tea available, each with its unique flavor profile and potential benefits. Try different varieties to find your favorites.

Enjoy it hot or cold: Green tea can be enjoyed both hot and cold, depending on your preference and the season.

Make it social: Share your love for green tea with friends and family by hosting a tea party or trying out new recipes together.

By incorporating these tips into your daily routine, you'll not only enjoy the delicious taste and numerous health benefits of green tea but also maximize its metabolism-boosting effects. So, raise your cup to a healthier, happier you!

Beyond the traditional cup, there's a world of possibilities for incorporating green tea's vibrant flavors and health benefits into your daily routine. For those seeking a culinary adventure, consider venturing into the realm of green tea-infused cuisine. Matcha, with its vibrant green hue and unique umami flavor, lends itself beautifully to both sweet and savory dishes. You can whisk it into salad dressings, sprinkle it over roasted vegetables, or even add a spoonful to your morning oatmeal for an extra boost of antioxidants.

Green tea's culinary versatility doesn't stop at matcha. Brewed green tea can be used to create flavorful marinades for meat or tofu, add depth to soups and stews, or even be used as a base for refreshing sorbet. The possibilities are truly endless, limited only by your imagination and culinary curiosity.

Incorporating green tea into your skincare routine is another delightful way to harness its antioxidant power. Green tea extracts are commonly found in facial cleansers, toners, moisturizers, and masks. These products can help protect your skin from free radical damage, reduce inflammation, and promote a youthful, radiant complexion. You can even try brewing a strong cup of green tea and using it as a facial toner or mist.

For a truly immersive green tea experience, consider exploring the world of green tea baths. In Japan, green tea baths are a traditional practice believed to promote relaxation, detoxification, and skin health. Simply add a few green tea bags or a handful of loose leaf tea to your bathwater and soak in the soothing aroma and therapeutic properties.

As you embark on your Green Tea Metabolism Makeover journey, remember that consistency is key. Make green tea a daily ritual, experimenting with different varieties, preparation methods, and culinary creations to keep things exciting. Embrace the versatility of this extraordinary beverage and allow it to become an integral part of your lifestyle.

By making green tea a cornerstone of your daily routine, you're not just enjoying a delicious drink; you're investing in your health, enhancing your metabolism, and setting the stage for a transformative journey towards a healthier, happier you.

Tracking Your Progress: Monitoring Your Weight Loss Journey

Embarking on any transformative journey, whether it's a physical makeover or a personal development quest, requires more than just setting a goal; it demands a keen awareness of your progress. The 28-Day Green Tea Metabolism Makeover is no exception. Tracking your progress isn't just about stepping on a scale; it's about understanding the subtle shifts in your body composition, energy levels, and overall well-being as you embrace the power of green tea. Think of it as charting your course on a map, ensuring you're headed in the right direction and making adjustments as needed to reach your ultimate destination: a healthier, more vibrant you.

Why is tracking your progress so crucial? First and foremost, it provides a tangible measure of your accomplishments, serving as a powerful motivator to keep you on track. Seeing the numbers on the scale decrease, your waistline shrink, or your body fat percentage drop can be incredibly rewarding and reinforcing. These small victories, when celebrated and acknowledged, fuel your determination and propel you forward on your weight loss journey.

Beyond motivation, tracking your progress offers valuable insights into how your body is responding to the Green Tea Metabolism Makeover plan. It allows you to identify what's working, what's not, and where adjustments might be necessary. For instance, if you notice your weight loss plateauing, you can analyze your food journal to identify potential areas for improvement, such as increasing your green tea intake, adjusting your meal portions, or incorporating more physical activity.

So, how do you effectively track your progress? There are several methods, each offering unique insights into your transformation.

Weighing Yourself: Stepping on the scale is perhaps the most common way to monitor weight loss progress. While it's important to remember that weight can fluctuate due to factors like water retention and muscle gain, regular weigh-ins can provide a general overview of your overall progress. Aim to weigh yourself at the same time each day, ideally in the morning after using the restroom and before eating or drinking.

Taking Body Measurements: Measuring your waist, hips, thighs, and arms can provide a more detailed picture of how your body composition is changing. Even if the scale doesn't budge, you might notice a decrease in inches, indicating a loss of body fat and an increase in lean muscle mass. Take your measurements at the beginning of the 28-day plan and then again every week or two to track your progress.

Monitoring Body Fat Percentage: Body fat percentage is a more accurate indicator of body composition than weight alone. It represents the proportion of your body weight that is composed of fat. You can measure your body fat percentage using various methods, such as skinfold calipers, bioelectrical impedance analysis (BIA) scales, or dual-energy X-ray absorptiometry (DEXA) scans. Consult with a healthcare professional or fitness expert to determine the most appropriate method for you.

Assessing Energy Levels and Mood: Pay attention to how you feel throughout the day. Are you experiencing more energy, better focus, and improved mood? These subjective measures can be just as important as objective data in gauging your overall well-being and the effectiveness of the Green Tea Metabolism Makeover plan.

Keeping a Food Journal: Recording your daily food intake, including green tea consumption, can provide valuable insights into your eating habits, portion sizes, and potential triggers for overeating or unhealthy choices. By analyzing your food journal, you can identify patterns, make adjustments, and ensure you're staying on track with the meal plan.

Tracking Exercise: Keep a record of your workouts, noting the type of exercise, duration, intensity, and how you felt afterward. This will help you monitor your progress, identify areas for improvement, and ensure you're getting enough physical activity to support your weight loss goals.

In addition to these objective measures, I encourage you to keep a journal to document your experiences, thoughts, and feelings throughout the 28-day journey. This journal can serve as a valuable tool for self-reflection, allowing you to track not only your physical changes but also your emotional and mental well-being.

As you write in your journal, consider the following prompts:

How do you feel after drinking green tea? Do you notice any changes in your energy levels, focus, or mood?

What challenges have you faced during the makeover, and how have you overcome them?

What are you most proud of so far?

What are your goals for the remainder of the 28 days?

How has green tea impacted your overall health and well-being?

Your journal can become a source of inspiration, motivation, and accountability. It can also serve as a reminder of how far you've come and the positive changes you've made in your life.

Remember, the Green Tea Metabolism Makeover is not just about reaching a specific number on the scale. It's about creating a sustainable lifestyle that supports your overall health and well-being. By tracking your progress, you'll gain valuable insights, stay motivated, and make informed decisions to ensure you achieve your goals and maintain your results long after the 28 days are over.

Chapter 4: Fueling Your Body: The Green Tea Metabolism Meal Plan

The foundation of the Green Tea Metabolism Makeover lies in a well-balanced diet, a nourishing symphony of flavors and nutrients that fuels your body's transformation. Think of your meals as a harmonious blend of ingredients, each playing a vital role in optimizing your metabolism, promoting satiety, and supporting overall health.

At the heart of this dietary symphony are macronutrients, the essential building blocks that provide your body with energy and support various physiological functions. The three primary macronutrients – protein, carbohydrates, and fats – each have unique roles to play in your weight loss journey.

Protein, often referred to as the "building block" of the body, is crucial for repairing and maintaining tissues, building muscle mass, and producing enzymes and hormones. When it comes to weight loss, protein takes center stage due to its ability to increase satiety, the feeling of fullness after a meal. Protein-rich foods take longer to digest than carbohydrates or fats, keeping you feeling satisfied and less likely to succumb to cravings between meals. Additionally, protein has a higher thermic effect of food (TEF), meaning your body burns more calories digesting and processing protein compared to other macronutrients.

Carbohydrates, the body's primary source of energy, fuel your brain, muscles, and other organs. However, not all carbohydrates are created equal. Simple carbohydrates, found in processed foods, sugary drinks, and refined grains, are quickly digested and can lead to blood sugar spikes and crashes, leaving you feeling tired and hungry. Complex carbohydrates, on the other hand, found in whole grains, legumes, fruits, and vegetables, provide sustained energy and are rich in fiber, which promotes digestive health and helps regulate blood sugar levels. Choosing complex carbohydrates over simple ones is key to maintaining stable energy levels, preventing cravings, and supporting your weight loss goals.

Fat, once demonized as a dietary villain, is now recognized as an essential nutrient with a multitude of benefits. Healthy fats, found in avocados, nuts, seeds, olive oil, and fatty fish, play a crucial role in hormone production, nutrient absorption, and cell membrane health. They also contribute to satiety, helping you feel full and satisfied after meals. However, it's important to distinguish between healthy fats and unhealthy fats. Unsaturated fats, like those found in olive oil and avocados, are considered heart-healthy and can help lower cholesterol levels. Saturated and trans fats, found in processed foods, fried foods, and baked goods, should be limited as they can raise cholesterol levels and increase the risk of heart disease.

While macronutrients provide energy, micronutrients, such as vitamins and minerals, are essential for countless bodily functions. These tiny but mighty nutrients act as co-factors in various metabolic processes, supporting everything from immune function and bone health to energy production and cognitive function. A deficiency in even one micronutrient can disrupt these processes and hinder your weight loss efforts.

Ensuring adequate micronutrient intake is as simple as filling your plate with a rainbow of colorful fruits and vegetables. Each color represents a different array of vitamins, minerals, and antioxidants that work synergistically to support your overall health and well-being. Incorporating green tea into your diet can further enhance your micronutrient intake, as it contains various vitamins and minerals, including vitamin C, vitamin K, and manganese.

Portion control and calorie density are two additional concepts that are crucial for successful weight management. Portion control involves being mindful of the amount of food you consume at each meal and snack. Even healthy foods can contribute to weight gain if eaten in excess. Calorie density, on the other hand, refers to the number of calories a food contains relative to its weight or volume.

Foods with low calorie density, such as fruits, vegetables, and whole grains, tend to be more filling and satisfying, allowing you to eat larger portions while consuming fewer calories.

To optimize your Green Tea Metabolism Makeover, focus on incorporating whole, unprocessed foods into your diet. These foods are typically lower in calories, sugar, and unhealthy fats, while being rich in nutrients, fiber, and antioxidants. Whole foods nourish your body with the essential vitamins, minerals, and phytochemicals it needs to function optimally and achieve your weight loss goals.

By prioritizing protein, complex carbohydrates, healthy fats, and a wide variety of fruits and vegetables, you'll create a dietary foundation that supports your metabolism, curbs cravings, and provides sustained energy throughout the day. Remember, a balanced diet is not about deprivation; it's about making informed choices and enjoying a diverse array of nutritious and delicious foods.

As you embark on this transformative journey, embrace the power of whole, unprocessed foods and allow them to nourish your body from the inside out. With each mindful bite, you're not just fueling your weight loss efforts; you're investing in your long-term health and well-being.

The Green Tea Metabolism Food Pyramid: Building Your Plate for Success

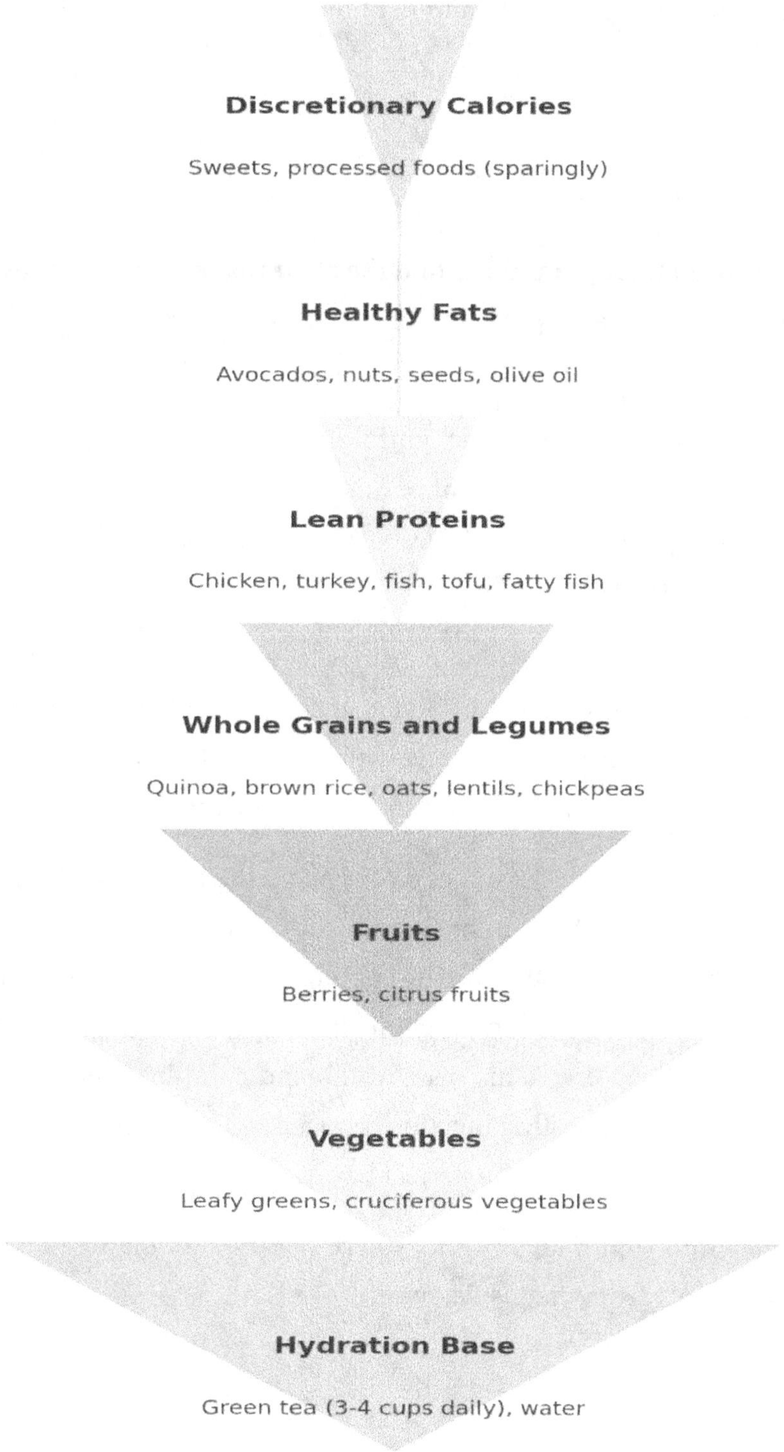

Discretionary Calories

Sweets, processed foods (sparingly)

Healthy Fats

Avocados, nuts, seeds, olive oil

Lean Proteins

Chicken, turkey, fish, tofu, fatty fish

Whole Grains and Legumes

Quinoa, brown rice, oats, lentils, chickpeas

Fruits

Berries, citrus fruits

Vegetables

Leafy greens, cruciferous vegetables

Hydration Base

Green tea (3-4 cups daily), water

Embarking on the Green Tea Metabolism Makeover is a journey toward a healthier, more vibrant you. At the heart of this transformation lies a balanced and nourishing diet, a symphony of flavors and nutrients that fuel your body's fat-burning potential and support your overall well-being. To guide you on this culinary adventure, we've crafted the Green Tea Metabolism Food Pyramid, a visual representation of the ideal food proportions for achieving your weight loss and metabolic goals.

The Foundation: Green Tea

At the base of this transformative pyramid, we find the elixir that sets our journey in motion: Green Tea. This revitalizing beverage, celebrated for centuries for its numerous health benefits, is the cornerstone of your metabolism makeover.

Each cup of green tea you enjoy isn't just a delightful drink; it's a potent dose of antioxidants and metabolism-boosting compounds like catechins and EGCG. These powerful substances work synergistically to increase your body's calorie-burning potential and enhance fat oxidation, contributing to a leaner, healthier you.

To maximize the benefits of green tea, aim to consume 3-4 cups throughout your day. Start your morning with a vibrant matcha latte, a creamy and energizing blend of matcha powder, milk, and a touch of sweetness. The earthy aroma and gentle caffeine of matcha will awaken your senses and provide a sustained energy boost without the jitters often associated with coffee.

As you transition into your workday, savor a cup of sencha, the most popular green tea in Japan. Its delicate balance of grassy notes, umami, and subtle sweetness offers a refreshing and invigorating experience. With a moderate caffeine content, sencha can help you maintain focus and productivity throughout the afternoon slump. As the day winds down, embrace the tranquility of a calming cup of chamomile green tea. This delightful blend combines the soothing properties of chamomile with the metabolism-boosting benefits of green tea. Chamomile has long been used to promote relaxation and sleep, making it the perfect beverage to unwind with before bed.

By integrating green tea into your daily routine, you're not only indulging in a delicious beverage but also nourishing your body from the inside out.

Building Blocks: Vegetables and Fruits

As we ascend the pyramid, a colorful array of vegetables and fruits awaits us. These vibrant treasures should fill half of your plate at each meal, providing a wealth of essential nutrients, fiber, and antioxidants. Imagine a rainbow of colors on your plate, each hue representing a unique combination of vitamins, minerals, and phytochemicals.

Embrace the dark, leafy embrace of spinach and kale, their high fiber content promoting satiety and supporting digestive health. Explore the cruciferous family – broccoli, cauliflower, Brussels sprouts, and cabbage – their sulfur-containing compounds aiding detoxification and potentially protecting against chronic diseases.

And don't forget the sweetness of nature's candy! Berries, citrus fruits, and apples offer a burst of flavor and essential nutrients without the added sugars of processed treats. Let their natural sweetness tantalize your taste buds while nourishing your body from the inside out.

Incorporate a variety of vegetables and fruits into your meals throughout the day. Start your day with a spinach and berry smoothie, enjoy a salad packed with colorful vegetables for lunch, and savor roasted vegetables as a side dish for dinner. The possibilities are endless, and the more variety you include, the more nutrients you'll reap.

The Foundation: Whole Grains and Legumes

Moving up the pyramid, we encounter the sturdy foundation of whole grains and legumes. These complex carbohydrates provide your body with sustained energy, releasing glucose slowly to fuel your activities throughout the day. Unlike their refined counterparts, whole grains and legumes retain their fiber-rich bran and germ, offering a wealth of nutrients and promoting digestive health.

Choose whole-grain bread, pasta, and rice over their refined versions, and embark on a culinary adventure with the nutty flavors of quinoa, brown rice, and farro. Lentils, chickpeas, black beans, and kidney beans are not only packed with protein but also offer a good source of fiber and iron. These fiber-rich options not only keep you feeling full and satisfied but also help regulate blood sugar levels, preventing energy crashes and cravings.

Building Blocks: Lean Protein

Next on our culinary journey, we arrive at the protein-packed domain of Lean Protein. These essential nutrients are the building blocks of your body, crucial for maintaining muscle mass and a healthy metabolism. Think of lean protein as the foundation for a strong and resilient body.

Incorporate sources like chicken, turkey, fish, tofu, beans, lentils, and eggs into your meals. These options provide a wealth of essential amino acids, the building blocks of protein, which support muscle growth, repair, and overall bodily functions. Aim to include a source of lean protein at every meal to ensure your body has the necessary building blocks for optimal health and metabolism.

As we ascend further, we reach the realm of Healthy Fats. Don't let the word "fat" scare you! These essential nutrients are crucial for hormone production, nutrient absorption, and maintaining the integrity of your cell membranes. They also contribute to satiety, helping you feel full and satisfied after meals.

Embrace the creamy goodness of avocados, a versatile fruit packed with heart-healthy monounsaturated fats, fiber, and a wealth of vitamins and minerals. Add slices to your salads, mash them into guacamole, or spread them on whole-grain toast for a satisfying and nutritious meal.

Savor the satisfying crunch of nuts and seeds, such as almonds, walnuts, chia seeds, and flaxseeds. These nutrient powerhouses are rich in healthy fats, protein, and fiber, making them a perfect snack or addition to your breakfast yogurt or oatmeal. Drizzle your salads and vegetables with extra virgin olive oil, a cornerstone of the Mediterranean diet, celebrated for its anti-inflammatory properties and potential heart-healthy benefits. And don't forget the omega-3 fatty acids found in fatty fish like salmon, tuna, and mackerel. These essential fats have been linked to numerous health benefits, including improved heart health, brain function, and mood.

While incorporating healthy fats is crucial, moderation is key. These fats are calorie-dense, so be mindful of your portion sizes to ensure you stay within your calorie goals. A small handful of nuts, a tablespoon of olive oil, or a 3-ounce serving of fatty fish are all reasonable portions that can provide your body with the healthy fats it needs without exceeding your calorie limits.

Finally, at the very top of our pyramid, we find the occasional Treats and Indulgences. While the majority of your diet should consist of whole, unprocessed foods, it's important to allow yourself some flexibility and enjoyment. Depriving yourself of all treats can lead to feelings of restriction and ultimately derail your progress.

Allow yourself to savor a small piece of dark chocolate, a naturally sweet and antioxidant-rich treat that can satisfy your sweet tooth without derailing your diet. Indulge in a fruit-infused yogurt parfait, a delicious and nutritious dessert that combines the sweetness of fruit with the protein and probiotics of yogurt. Or enjoy a homemade granola bar made with whole ingredients like oats, nuts, seeds, and dried fruits.

Remember, these treats should be enjoyed in moderation and should not replace the nutrient-dense foods that form the foundation of the Green Tea Metabolism Food Pyramid. Aim for a balance that allows you to enjoy the pleasures of food while still nourishing your body and supporting your weight loss goals.

By understanding the role of each food group and incorporating green tea as a cornerstone, you'll be well on your way to achieving a healthier, leaner, and more energized you. Remember, the Green Tea Metabolism Food Pyramid is not just a guide; it's a transformative tool that empowers you to make informed choices and create a sustainable and enjoyable way of eating. With each meal, you're not just fueling your body; you're investing in your long-term health and well-being. So, let this pyramid be your compass as you navigate the delicious and nutritious world of whole foods and green tea.

Delicious and Nutritious Green Tea Recipes: Adding Flavor to Your Meals

1. Matcha Overnight Oats:

Ingredients:

- ½ cup rolled oats (use certified gluten-free if needed)
- 2 tsp chia seeds
- 1 tsp matcha powder
- ½ tsp cinnamon (optional)
- Pinch of salt
- 1 cup plain Greek yogurt or dairy-free alternative
- 1 cup unsweetened milk of choice (almond, oat, etc.)
- 1 tsp vanilla extract
- 1-2 tsp maple syrup or honey (adjust to taste)
- Toppings: berries, sliced banana, nuts, seeds, etc.

Instructions:

1. In a jar or container, combine oats, chia seeds, matcha, cinnamon, and salt.

2. Add yogurt, milk, vanilla, and sweetener. Stir well until combined.

3. Cover and refrigerate for at least 2 hours or overnight.

4. Before serving, stir and add desired toppings. Enjoy cold or gently warmed.

Green Tea Smoothie Bowl:

Ingredients:

- 1 cup brewed and cooled green tea
- 1 frozen banana
- ½ cup frozen mango chunks
- 1 cup fresh spinach
- ¼ avocado (optional, for creaminess)
- Toppings: berries, sliced kiwi, coconut flakes, granola, etc.

Instructions:

1. Combine all ingredients in a blender and blend until smooth and creamy.

2. Pour into a bowl and decorate with desired toppings.

Green Tea Eggs (Ajitsuke Tamago):

Ingredients:

- 6 hard-boiled eggs
- 1 cup brewed green tea
- ½ cup soy sauce
- ¼ cup mirin (sweet rice wine)
- 1 star anise
- 1 cinnamon stick
- 2 cloves garlic, peeled and lightly smashed

Instructions:

1. Gently crack the shells of the hard-boiled eggs all over.

2. In a saucepan, combine the remaining ingredients and bring to a simmer.

3. Add the eggs and simmer for at least 1 hour, or up to 4 hours for a stronger flavor.

4. Let the eggs cool completely in the liquid before peeling and serving.

Matcha Pancakes:

Ingredients:

- 1 cup all-purpose flour (use gluten-free blend if needed)
- 2 tbsp sugar
- 2 tsp baking powder
- ½ tsp salt
- 1 cup milk
- 1 egg
- 2 tbsp melted butter
- 1 tsp matcha powder

Instructions:

1. Whisk together flour, sugar, baking powder, and salt.

2. In a separate bowl, whisk together milk, egg, melted butter, and matcha powder.

3. Pour the wet ingredients into the dry ingredients and whisk until just combined.

4. Heat a lightly oiled griddle or frying pan over medium heat.

5. Pour ¼ cup of batter onto the griddle for each pancake.

6. Cook until bubbles form on the surface, then flip and cook until golden brown.

7. Serve with your favorite toppings like fruit and maple syrup.

Green Tea Chia Seed Pudding:

Ingredients:

- 1 cup brewed and cooled green tea
- ¼ cup chia seeds
- 2 tbsp sweetener of choice (maple syrup, honey, agave)
- ½ tsp vanilla extract (optional)
- Toppings: berries, chopped nuts, shredded coconut

Instructions:

1. In a jar or container, combine green tea, chia seeds, sweetener, and vanilla extract (if using).

2. Stir well to ensure the chia seeds are evenly distributed.

3. Cover and refrigerate for at least 4 hours or overnight, until thickened.

4. Before serving, stir and add desired toppings.

Lunch

Green Tea Salmon Salad:

Ingredients:

- 12 oz cooked salmon, flaked
- 4 cups mixed greens (arugula, spinach, romaine)
- ½ cup cucumber, diced
- ½ cup cherry tomatoes, halved
- ¼ cup red onion, thinly sliced
- 2 tbsp chopped fresh dill
- Green Tea Vinaigrette:
- ¼ cup extra virgin olive oil
- 2 tbsp lemon juice
- 1 tbsp Dijon mustard
- 1 tsp honey or maple syrup
- ½ tsp matcha powder
- Salt and pepper to taste

Instructions:

In a large bowl, combine the salmon, mixed greens, cucumber, tomatoes, red onion, and dill.

In a small bowl, whisk together the vinaigrette ingredients until emulsified.

Drizzle the vinaigrette over the salad and toss gently to combine.

Serve immediately.

Matcha Hummus:

Ingredients:

- 1 can (15 oz) chickpeas, rinsed and drained
- ¼ cup tahini
- 2 tbsp lemon juice
- 2 tbsp olive oil
- 1 clove garlic, minced
- 1 tsp matcha powder
- Salt and pepper to taste
- Optional: a pinch of ground cumin or smoked paprika

Instructions:

Combine all ingredients in a food processor or blender.

Process until smooth and creamy, scraping down the sides as needed.

Adjust seasonings to taste.

Serve with whole-wheat pita bread, vegetables, or crackers.

Green Tea Noodle Salad:

Ingredients:

- 8 oz soba noodles (buckwheat noodles)
- 1 cup shredded carrots
- 1 cup shredded red cabbage
- ½ cup chopped cucumber
- ½ cup shelled edamame

- ¼ cup chopped fresh cilantro
- Green Tea Dressing:
- ¼ cup rice vinegar
- 2 tbsp soy sauce
- 1 tbsp sesame oil
- 1 tbsp honey or maple syrup
- 1 tsp grated ginger
- ½ tsp matcha powder

Instructions:

Cook soba noodles according to package directions. Rinse under cold water and drain.

In a large bowl, combine the noodles with carrots, cabbage, cucumber, edamame, and cilantro.

In a small bowl, whisk together the dressing ingredients until combined.

Pour the dressing over the salad and toss to coat.

Serve chilled.

Green Tea Chicken Salad:

Ingredients:

- 2 cups cooked chicken, shredded
- 1 cup celery, chopped
- ½ cup grapes, halved
- ½ cup walnuts, chopped
- Green Tea Mayonnaise Dressing:
- ½ cup mayonnaise
- 2 tbsp lemon juice
- 1 tbsp chopped fresh chives
- 1 tsp matcha powder
- Salt and pepper to taste

Instructions:

In a large bowl, combine the chicken, celery, grapes, and walnuts.

In a small bowl, whisk together the dressing ingredients until combined.

Add the dressing to the chicken mixture and toss to coat.

Serve on whole-wheat bread, lettuce wraps, or crackers.

Green Tea Lentil Soup:

Ingredients:

- 1 tbsp olive oil
- 1 onion, chopped
- 2 cloves garlic, minced
- 1 tsp curry powder
- ½ tsp ground cumin
- ½ tsp turmeric
- 4 cups vegetable broth
- 1 cup red lentils
- 1 can (14 oz) diced tomatoes
- 1 cup chopped carrots
- 1 cup chopped kale or spinach
- ½ cup brewed green tea
- Salt and pepper to taste
- Optional: a dollop of plain yogurt or coconut milk for serving

Instructions:

Heat olive oil in a large pot over medium heat. Add onion and cook until softened.

Add garlic, curry powder, cumin, and turmeric and cook for 1 minute more.

Add broth, lentils, tomatoes, carrots, and kale or spinach. Bring to a boil, then reduce heat and simmer for 20-25 minutes or until lentils are tender.

Stir in green tea and season with salt and pepper to taste.

Serve hot, with a dollop of yogurt or coconut milk if desired.

Dinner:

Green Tea Glazed Salmon:

Ingredients:

- 4 salmon fillets (6 oz each)
- ¼ cup soy sauce (use tamari for gluten-free)
- 2 tbsp honey
- 1 tbsp grated ginger
- 2 tbsp brewed green tea
- 1 tbsp sesame oil
- Salt and pepper to taste

Instructions:

1. In a shallow dish, whisk together soy sauce, honey, ginger, green tea, and sesame oil.

2. Place salmon fillets in the marinade and turn to coat.

3. Marinate for at least 30 minutes or up to 2 hours in the refrigerator.

4. Preheat oven to 400°F (200°C) or prepare a grill.

5. Place salmon on a baking sheet or grill grate.

6. Bake for 12-15 minutes or grill for 6-8 minutes per side, until cooked through.

7. Baste with remaining marinade during cooking.

8. Serve with steamed vegetables or a side salad.

Matcha Pesto Pasta:

Ingredients:

- 8 oz pasta (use gluten-free pasta if needed)
- 2 cups packed fresh basil leaves
- ¼ cup pine nuts (or walnuts)
- 2 cloves garlic
- ¼ cup grated Parmesan cheese (omit for vegan)
- ½ tsp matcha powder
- ¼ cup extra virgin olive oil
- Salt and pepper to taste

Instructions:

1. Cook pasta according to package directions.

2. While pasta cooks, combine basil, pine nuts, garlic, Parmesan (if using), matcha, and olive oil in a food processor or blender.

3. Process until smooth, adding more olive oil if needed for desired consistency.

4. Season with salt and pepper to taste.

5. Drain pasta and toss with pesto.

6. Serve warm with additional Parmesan and fresh basil leaves (if using).

Green Tea Chicken Stir-Fry:

Ingredients:

- 1 lb boneless, skinless chicken breasts, cut into strips
- 1 tbsp cornstarch
- 1 tbsp soy sauce (use tamari for gluten-free)
- 1 tbsp sesame oil
- 1 onion, sliced
- 1 bell pepper (any color), sliced
- 1 cup broccoli florets
- ½ cup snow peas

Green Tea Stir-Fry Sauce:

- ¼ cup brewed green tea
- 2 tbsp soy sauce (use tamari for gluten-free)
- 1 tbsp honey
- 1 tbsp rice vinegar
- 1 tsp grated ginger
- ½ tsp minced garlic
- Optional: garnish with chopped green onions and sesame seeds

Instructions:

1. In a bowl, combine chicken with cornstarch and soy sauce.

2. Heat sesame oil in a large skillet or wok over medium-high heat. Add chicken and cook until browned on all sides. Remove from skillet.

3. Add vegetables to the skillet and stir-fry until crisp-tender.

4. In a small bowl, whisk together stir-fry sauce ingredients.

5. Return chicken to the skillet and add the sauce. Stir-fry until sauce thickens and chicken is cooked through.

6. Serve over brown rice or quinoa.

Matcha Tofu Scramble:

Ingredients:

- 1 block (14 oz) extra firm tofu, crumbled
- 1 tbsp olive oil
- ½ onion, chopped
- 1 bell pepper (any color), chopped
- 1 cup mushrooms, sliced
- 1 tsp turmeric
- ½ tsp garlic powder
- ½ tsp onion powder
- ¼ tsp black pepper
- 1 tsp matcha powder
- Salt to taste
- Optional: nutritional yeast, chopped chives, hot sauce

Instructions:

1. Heat olive oil in a large skillet over medium heat.

2. Add onion and bell pepper and cook until softened.

3. Add mushrooms and cook until browned.

4. Add crumbled tofu and spices (turmeric, garlic powder, onion powder, black pepper, matcha, salt). Cook, stirring frequently, until heated through.

5. Serve warm with avocado, whole-wheat toast, or a side salad.

Green Tea Veggie Curry:

Ingredients:

- 1 tbsp olive oil
- 1 onion, chopped
- 2 cloves garlic, minced
- 1 tbsp curry powder
- ½ tsp ground cumin
- ½ tsp ground coriander
- ¼ tsp cayenne pepper
- 1 can (14 oz) coconut milk
- 1 cup vegetable broth
- 2 cups mixed vegetables (broccoli, cauliflower, carrots, potatoes, etc.)
- ½ cup brewed green tea
- Salt and pepper to taste
- Optional: a squeeze of lime juice and chopped cilantro for serving

Instructions:

1. Heat olive oil in a large pot over medium heat. Add onion and cook until softened.

2. Add garlic, curry powder, cumin, coriander, and cayenne pepper and cook for 1 minute more.

3. Add coconut milk, broth, and vegetables. Bring to a boil, then reduce heat and simmer until vegetables are tender, about 15-20 minutes.

4. Stir in green tea and season with salt and pepper to taste.

5. Serve over brown rice or quinoa, with a squeeze of lime juice and chopped cilantro if desired.

Snacks:

Matcha Energy Bites:

Ingredients:

- 1 cup pitted dates
- ½ cup raw almonds
- ½ cup raw cashews
- ¼ cup shredded coconut
- 2 tbsp matcha powder
- Pinch of salt

Instructions:

1. In a food processor, combine all ingredients and pulse until a sticky dough forms. If the mixture seems too dry, add a tablespoon of water at a time until the desired consistency is reached.

2. Roll the dough into small balls (about 1 tablespoon each).

3. Place the energy bites on a baking sheet lined with parchment paper and refrigerate for at least 30 minutes to firm up.

4. Store in an airtight container in the refrigerator for up to 1 week.

Green Tea Yogurt Bark:

Ingredients:

- 2 cups plain Greek yogurt (or dairy-free alternative)
- 1 tbsp honey or maple syrup
- 1 tsp matcha powder
- ½ cup mixed berries (blueberries, raspberries, strawberries)
- ¼ cup granola
- ¼ cup chopped nuts (almonds, walnuts, pecans)

Instructions:

1. Line a baking sheet with parchment paper.

2. In a bowl, combine yogurt, honey, and matcha powder. Stir until smooth and well combined.

3. Spread the yogurt mixture evenly onto the prepared baking sheet, creating a thin layer.

4. Sprinkle the berries, granola, and nuts evenly over the yogurt.

5. Freeze for at least 2 hours, or until completely firm.

6. Break the bark into pieces and enjoy as a refreshing and healthy snack.

Green Tea Popcorn:

Ingredients:

- ½ cup popcorn kernels
- 1 tbsp coconut oil
- 1 green tea bag (or 1 tsp loose leaf green tea)
- Salt to taste

Instructions:

1. In a large pot with a lid, heat the coconut oil over medium heat.

2. Add the popcorn kernels and cover the pot.

3. Shake the pot occasionally until the popping slows down.

4. Remove from heat and transfer the popcorn to a large bowl.

5. Meanwhile, brew a strong cup of green tea. If using a tea bag, remove it. If using loose leaf tea, strain the leaves.

6. Drizzle the brewed green tea over the popcorn and toss to coat evenly.

7. Sprinkle with salt to taste.

8. Let cool slightly before serving.

Desserts:

Matcha Ice Cream:

Ingredients:

- 1 can (14 oz) full-fat coconut milk
- ½ cup sweetener of choice (maple syrup, honey, agave)
- 2 tbsp matcha powder
- Pinch of salt

Instructions:

1. In a blender, combine all ingredients and blend until smooth and well combined.

2. If using an ice cream maker, pour the mixture into the ice cream maker and churn according to the manufacturer's instructions.

3. If you don't have an ice cream maker, pour the mixture into a freezer-safe container and freeze for at least 4 hours, stirring every hour to prevent ice crystals from forming.

Green Tea Chocolate Truffles:

Ingredients:

- 4 oz dark chocolate, finely chopped
- ¼ cup full-fat coconut milk
- 1 tbsp matcha powder
- 1 tsp coconut oil
- Optional toppings: chopped nuts, shredded coconut, matcha powder

Instructions:

1. Place the chopped chocolate in a heatproof bowl.

2. In a saucepan, heat the coconut milk over low heat until hot but not boiling.

3. Pour the hot coconut milk over the chocolate and let it sit for a few minutes to melt.

4. Add the matcha powder and coconut oil to the chocolate mixture and whisk until smooth and well combined.

5. Pour the mixture into a shallow dish lined with parchment paper.

6. Refrigerate for at least 2 hours, or until firm.

7. Once firm, use a spoon to scoop out small portions of the mixture and roll them into balls.

8. Roll the truffles in desired toppings, if using.

9. Store in an airtight container in the refrigerator for up to 1 week.

Matcha Energy Bites:

Ingredients:

- 1 cup pitted dates
- ½ cup raw almonds
- ½ cup raw cashews
- ¼ cup shredded coconut
- 2 tbsp matcha powder
- Pinch of salt

Instructions:

In a food processor, combine all ingredients and pulse until a sticky dough forms. If the mixture seems too dry, add a tablespoon of water at a time until the desired consistency is reached.

Roll the dough into small balls (about 1 tablespoon each).

Place the energy bites on a baking sheet lined with parchment paper and refrigerate for at least 30 minutes to firm up.

Store in an airtight container in the refrigerator for up to 1 week.

Green Tea Yogurt Bark:

Ingredients:

- 2 cups plain Greek yogurt (or dairy-free alternative)
- 1 tbsp honey or maple syrup
- 1 tsp matcha powder
- ½ cup mixed berries (blueberries, raspberries, strawberries)
- ¼ cup granola
- ¼ cup chopped nuts (almonds, walnuts, pecans)

Instructions:

Line a baking sheet with parchment paper.

In a bowl, combine yogurt, honey, and matcha powder. Stir until smooth and well combined.

Spread the yogurt mixture evenly onto the prepared baking sheet, creating a thin layer.

Sprinkle the berries, granola, and nuts evenly over the yogurt.

Freeze for at least 2 hours, or until completely firm.

Break the bark into pieces and enjoy as a refreshing and healthy snack.

Green Tea Popcorn:

Ingredients:

- ½ cup popcorn kernels
- 1 tbsp coconut oil
- 1 green tea bag (or 1 tsp loose leaf green tea)
- Salt to taste

Instructions:

In a large pot with a lid, heat the coconut oil over medium heat.

Add the popcorn kernels and cover the pot.

Shake the pot occasionally until the popping slows down.

Remove from heat and transfer the popcorn to a large bowl.

Meanwhile, brew a strong cup of green tea. If using a tea bag, remove it. If using loose leaf tea, strain the leaves.

Drizzle the brewed green tea over the popcorn and toss to coat evenly.

Sprinkle with salt to taste.

Let cool slightly before serving.

Green Tea Enthusiasts, Your Voice Matters!

Hey there, wellness warrior in the making!

I hope "The Green Tea Metabolism Makeover" has ignited your passion for a healthier lifestyle and fueled your journey towards a more vibrant you.

Now, I'm turning to you, the heart of the green tea community. Your experiences, insights, and triumphs on this 28-day journey are incredibly valuable. By sharing your honest thoughts in a review on Amazon, you're not only helping other health-conscious individuals discover the transformative power of green tea, but you're also shaping the future of holistic wellness.

Your feedback fuels my creativity and inspires me to continue crafting resources that empower you to become the best version of yourself. Whether you've mastered a new green tea recipe, conquered a challenging workout, or simply found inner peace through mindful eating, your review makes a difference.

How to Share Your 5-Star Transformation Story on Amazon:

1. Visit the Amazon page for "The Green Tea Metabolism Makeover."
2. Scroll down to the "Customer Reviews" section.
3. Click on the "Write a customer review" button.
4. Give the book a well-deserved 5-star rating and share your inspiring transformation story!

It's that simple! Your voice matters, and together, we can make the green tea community even stronger and more vibrant.

Thank you for being a part of this transformative adventure!

Evelyn Green (Author of "The Green Tea Metabolism Makeover")

BONUS

HERE IS YOUR **BONUS**

[CLICK THE LINK TO GET YOUR BONUS]

OR SCAN THE QR CODE TO GET YOUR BONUS

Chapter 5: The Green Tea Workout: Exercising for Optimal Fat Burning

In our pursuit of a healthier, more vibrant life, we often focus on the external transformation shedding those extra pounds and sculpting a leaner physique. But the true magic of exercise lies in its ability to ignite a transformation that goes far beyond the mirror. It's about empowering your body from the inside out, strengthening your heart, building resilient muscles, fortifying your bones, and bolstering your defenses against chronic diseases.

Imagine your body as a symphony orchestra, each instrument playing a vital role in creating a harmonious melody of health and well-being. Exercise is the conductor's baton, orchestrating a symphony of physiological responses that enhance your cardiovascular health, fortify your muscles, increase bone density, and reduce the risk of chronic diseases.

Let's begin with the heart, the maestro of this intricate symphony. Regular exercise, particularly aerobic activities like brisk walking, running, swimming, or dancing, is a cardiovascular elixir. It strengthens your heart muscle, improves blood flow, and lowers blood pressure, reducing the risk of heart disease, stroke, and other cardiovascular ailments. Imagine your heart as a powerful pump, working tirelessly to deliver oxygen and nutrients to every cell in your body. Exercise trains this pump to become more efficient, ensuring optimal blood flow and reducing the strain on your cardiovascular system.

But the benefits of exercise don't stop at your heart. Your muscles, the unsung heroes of metabolism, are also profoundly impacted by regular physical activity. Strength training, whether through lifting weights, using resistance bands, or engaging in bodyweight exercises, stimulates muscle growth and strengthens existing muscle fibers. This not only enhances your physical appearance but also increases your basal metabolic rate (BMR), the number of calories your body burns at rest. In essence, building muscle turns your body into a more efficient calorie-burning machine, helping you shed pounds and maintain a healthy weight.

Beyond aesthetics and metabolism, strong muscles are essential for functional fitness, making everyday activities easier and reducing the risk of injuries. They also play a crucial role in maintaining good posture, supporting your joints, and preventing chronic pain. So, embrace the power of strength training and sculpt a body that is not only beautiful but also resilient and functional.

As we continue our exploration of exercise's benefits, we arrive at the skeletal system, the framework that supports our bodies and enables movement. Regular exercise, particularly weight-bearing activities like walking, running, and jumping, stimulates the production of new bone tissue and increases bone density. This is especially crucial for women, who are at higher risk of osteoporosis, a condition characterized by weakened bones and increased fracture risk. By engaging in weight-bearing exercise, you're not just building stronger muscles; you're also fortifying your bones and reducing your risk of fractures and falls.

But the benefits of exercise don't stop at your bones. This powerful lifestyle intervention has been shown to reduce the risk of numerous chronic diseases, including type 2 diabetes, certain types of cancer, and even Alzheimer's disease. Regular physical activity can improve insulin sensitivity, making it easier for your body to utilize glucose for energy and reducing the risk of insulin resistance, a major contributor to type 2 diabetes. Exercise can also bolster your immune system, enhance your mood, and improve your sleep quality, all of which contribute to a healthier and happier life.

Now, let's delve into the fascinating synergy between exercise and green tea, a dynamic duo that can amplify the effects of your metabolism makeover. Green tea, with its metabolism-boosting catechins and caffeine, has been shown to enhance the fat-burning effects of exercise. Studies suggest that consuming green tea before a workout can increase fat oxidation, meaning your body will utilize more stored fat for energy during exercise. This not only helps you shed pounds but also improves your exercise performance and endurance.

Moreover, green tea's antioxidant prowess comes to the forefront during exercise. As your body works harder, it generates free radicals, unstable molecules that can damage cells and tissues. Green tea's catechins, particularly EGCG, act as potent antioxidants, neutralizing these free radicals and protecting your cells from oxidative stress. This not only reduces muscle damage and inflammation but also supports faster recovery, allowing you to bounce back quicker and train more consistently.

Beyond the metabolic boost and antioxidant protection, green tea offers an array of other benefits that enhance your exercise experience. The gentle caffeine content in green tea provides a natural energy lift, increasing alertness, focus, and endurance during your workouts. Unlike the jittery energy from coffee, the L-theanine in green tea promotes a calm and focused state, allowing you to push through those challenging sets and reps.

Furthermore, green tea's hydrating properties can help replenish fluids lost during exercise, preventing dehydration and maintaining optimal performance. While plain water is essential for hydration, green tea offers the added benefits of antioxidants and electrolytes, which can aid in muscle function and recovery.

The 28-day Green Tea Metabolism Makeover plan recognizes the synergistic power of exercise and green tea, strategically incorporating both into a comprehensive lifestyle transformation. By enjoying green tea before, during, or after your workouts, you'll maximize its fat-burning, antioxidant, and energizing effects, while reaping the numerous benefits of exercise for your overall health and well-being.

As you embark on this transformative journey, embrace the power of movement and allow exercise to become an integral part of your daily routine. Whether it's a brisk walk in the park, a heart-pumping dance class, or a strength training session at the gym, find activities that you enjoy and that fit seamlessly into your lifestyle. Remember, consistency is key, so aim for at least 30 minutes of moderate-intensity exercise most days of the week.

But exercise isn't just about structured workouts; it's about embracing an active lifestyle. Take the stairs instead of the elevator, walk or bike to work, and find opportunities to move your body throughout the day. By incorporating these small changes, you'll not only increase your daily calorie expenditure but also improve your mood, reduce stress, and enhance your overall quality of life.

The Green Tea Workout Plan: Combining Cardio and Strength Training

When I first started my own journey towards a healthier lifestyle, I was overwhelmed by the sheer number of workout plans and exercise routines available. I tried everything from high-intensity interval training to yoga, but nothing seemed to stick. I felt lost and discouraged until I discovered the power of combining cardio and strength training in a balanced and sustainable way. The results were transformative, not only for my physique but also for my energy levels, mood, and overall well-being.

Now, I'm excited to share with you a Green Tea Workout Plan that incorporates the best of both worlds: cardiovascular exercise to get your heart pumping and burn calories, and strength training to build muscle and boost your metabolism. This plan is designed to be flexible and adaptable to your fitness level, whether you're a beginner just starting or a seasoned fitness enthusiast looking for a new challenge.

The Green Tea Metabolism Workout Plan: Your Path to a Stronger, Leaner You

This dynamic workout plan is designed to harness the synergistic power of green tea and exercise, maximizing fat burning and promoting overall health and well-being. Whether you're a beginner or a seasoned fitness enthusiast, this plan offers modifications and challenges to suit your individual needs and preferences. Remember to consult with your doctor before starting any new workout routine.

Monday: Kickstart Your Metabolism

- **Warm-up (5 minutes):** Begin with light cardio, such as brisk walking or jogging in place, followed by dynamic stretches like arm circles, leg swings, and torso twists.
- **Cardio (30 minutes):**
  - **Beginner:** Brisk walk for 30 minutes at a pace that elevates your heart rate but allows you to hold a conversation.
  - **Intermediate:** Jog for 20 minutes, alternating between a moderate pace and short bursts of faster running.
  - **Advanced:** Run for 30 minutes, incorporating hills or intervals to challenge your cardiovascular system.

- **Strength Training (30 minutes):**
  - 3 sets of 10-12 repetitions of each exercise:
    - **Squats:** Stand with feet shoulder-width apart, lower your body as if sitting in a chair, keeping your back straight and knees in line with your toes.
    - **Lunges:** Step forward with one leg and lower your body until both knees are bent at a 90-degree angle. Keep your front knee directly above your ankle.
    - **Push-ups:** Start in a plank position with hands shoulder-width apart. Lower your body until your chest nearly touches the floor, then push back up. Modify by doing push-ups on your knees if needed.
    - **Plank:** Hold a push-up position with forearms on the ground and body in a straight line from head to heels. Engage your core muscles and hold for 30-60 seconds.
- **Cool-down (5 minutes):** Gentle stretching to improve flexibility and prevent muscle soreness.

Tuesday: Active Recovery and Flexibility

- **Yoga or Pilates (30-45 minutes):** Choose a beginner-friendly class or follow an online video. Focus on poses that stretch your muscles and promote relaxation.
- **Foam Rolling (15 minutes):** Use a foam roller to massage your muscles and release tension. Focus on areas that feel tight or sore.

Wednesday: Pedal Power

- **Warm-up (5 minutes):** Light cardio, such as marching in place or high knees, followed by dynamic stretches.
- **Cycling (30-45 minutes):**
  - **Beginner:** Cycle at a moderate pace on flat terrain.
  - **Intermediate:** Incorporate intervals of higher intensity, such as sprinting for 30 seconds followed by 1 minute of rest.
  - **Advanced:** Add hills or increase resistance for a more challenging workout.
- **Cool-down (5 minutes):** Slow down your pace and stretch your legs and back.

Thursday: Upper Body Strength
- **Warm-up (5 minutes):** Light cardio and dynamic stretches, focusing on the upper body.
- **Strength Training (30 minutes):**
  - 3 sets of 10-12 repetitions of each exercise:
    - **Dumbbell Rows:** Hinge at your hips and pull a dumbbell towards your chest, squeezing your shoulder blade.
    - shoulder-width apart and press dumbbells straight up overhead.
    -
    - **Bicep Curls:** Curl dumbbells towards your shoulders, keeping your elbows close to your sides.

- **Tricep Dips:** Use a chair or bench to lower your body, bending at the elbows until your arms are at a 90-degree angle.
- **Cool-down (5 minutes):** Stretch your arms, shoulders, and back.

Friday: Full-Body Blast

- **Warm-up (5 minutes):** Light cardio and dynamic stretches for the whole body.
- **HIIT (20 minutes):**
  - Alternate between 30 seconds of high-intensity exercise and 30 seconds of rest for a total of 20 minutes.
  - Choose exercises like jumping jacks, burpees, mountain climbers, high knees, or sprints.
- **Strength Training (20 minutes):**
  - 2 sets of 15-20 repetitions of each exercise:
    - Squats
    - Lunges
    - Push-ups
    - Dumbbell rows
    - Plank (hold for 30-60 seconds)
- **Cool-down (5 minutes):** Full-body stretches to improve flexibility and prevent muscle soreness.

Weekend: Rest and Active Recovery

- **Restorative Yoga (30-45 minutes):** Focus on gentle stretches and poses that promote relaxation and recovery.
- **Light Cardio (30 minutes):** Enjoy a leisurely walk, swim, or bike ride.
-
- **Foam Rolling (15 minutes):** Use a foam roller to massage your muscles and release tension.

This detailed workout plan is your blueprint for success in the Green Tea Metabolism Makeover. Remember, consistency is key, so strive to stick to this schedule as closely as possible. Listen to your body and adjust the intensity or duration of your workouts as needed. And most importantly, have fun with it! Exercise should be an enjoyable part of your lifestyle, not a chore.

In my early attempts to establish a consistent exercise routine, I faced countless obstacles. My schedule felt jam-packed, motivation waxed and waned, and I often found excuses to skip workouts. Sound familiar? If you've ever struggled to make exercise a habit, you're not alone.

One of the most common barriers to exercise is the ever-present "lack of time." Between work, family commitments, and social obligations, carving out time for exercise can feel like an insurmountable challenge. But here's the secret: you don't need hours in the gym to reap the benefits of movement. Even short bursts of activity throughout the day can make a significant difference. Instead of viewing exercise as a monolithic block of time, break it down into smaller, more manageable chunks. A brisk 10-minute walk during your lunch break, a quick yoga session before bed, or even a few sets of squats and lunges while waiting for dinner to cook can all contribute to your daily activity goals. Remember, every minute of movement counts!

Another common hurdle is a lack of motivation. It's easy to feel uninspired or discouraged, especially when starting a new exercise routine. But motivation is not a constant; it fluctuates like the tides. The key is to find ways to reignite your spark when it starts to dim.

One of the most effective strategies is to find a workout buddy. Having someone to exercise with can provide accountability, encouragement, and a sense of camaraderie. You can challenge each other, celebrate each other's successes, and make exercise a fun social activity. If you don't have a friend or family member who shares your fitness goals, consider joining a group fitness class or finding a virtual workout buddy online.

Setting realistic goals is another crucial aspect of staying motivated. Instead of aiming for drastic changes overnight, focus on small, achievable goals that you can build upon over time. For example, instead of vowing to run a marathon in a month, start with a goal of walking for 30 minutes three times a week. As you achieve these smaller goals, you'll gain confidence and momentum, propelling you towards even greater achievements.

Celebrating your progress is equally important. Reward yourself for reaching your fitness milestones, whether it's a new workout outfit, a massage, or a guilt-free indulgence. These rewards not only reinforce positive behavior but also make the journey more enjoyable and sustainable.

In addition to these strategies, there are countless ways to make exercise more fun and engaging. Explore different activities until you find something you genuinely enjoy. If you dread the treadmill, try dancing, swimming, hiking, or rock climbing. The key is to find movement that brings you joy and makes you want to move.

Creating a playlist of your favorite upbeat music can also make your workouts more enjoyable. Music has been shown to improve mood, reduce perceived exertion, and increase motivation, making it the perfect companion for your sweat sessions.

Gamifying your workouts can also add an element of fun and competition. Set challenges for yourself, track your progress, and compete with friends or family members. There are numerous fitness apps and wearable devices that can help you track your activity, set goals, and earn rewards for your achievements.

Remember, the journey to a healthier, fitter you is not a sprint; it's a marathon. It's about making sustainable lifestyle changes that you can maintain for the long haul. By overcoming common barriers, setting realistic goals, and finding ways to make exercise enjoyable, you'll be well on your way to transforming your body, boosting your metabolism, and achieving lasting results.

Embrace the power of movement, and let it become an integral part of your daily life. Whether it's a morning yoga session, a lunchtime walk, or an evening bike ride, find ways to move your body that bring you joy and fulfillment. Remember, every step you take, every rep you complete, and every drop of sweat you shed is a victory on your path to a healthier, happier you.

Chapter 6: Stress Less, Weigh Less: The Mind-Body Connection and Weight Loss

A few years ago, I found myself caught in a whirlwind of stress. Work deadlines were piling up, family responsibilities were demanding my attention, and my once healthy lifestyle had fallen by the wayside. As the stress mounted, I noticed a disturbing trend: my jeans were getting tighter, and my energy levels were plummeting. Despite my best efforts to eat healthy and exercise, the scale refused to budge. I felt frustrated and defeated until I delved deeper into the intricate connection between stress and weight gain. What I discovered was a revelation that changed the way I approached my health and well-being.

Stress, while a natural part of life, can wreak havoc on our bodies in ways we may not realize. When we experience stress, our bodies initiate a cascade of physiological responses designed to help us cope with the perceived threat. This "fight-or-flight" response triggers the release of stress hormones like cortisol, adrenaline, and norepinephrine, which prepare our bodies for action.

In the short term, this stress response can be beneficial, providing us with the energy and focus we need to navigate challenging situations. However, when stress becomes chronic, these hormones can linger in our bodies, disrupting our metabolism and contributing to weight gain.

Cortisol, in particular, plays a central role in the stress-weight connection. This hormone, often dubbed the "stress hormone," is produced by the adrenal glands in response to stress. Its primary function is to increase blood sugar levels, providing our bodies with a quick source of energy to fuel our fight-or-flight response. However, when cortisol levels remain elevated for prolonged periods, it can lead to a host of metabolic disturbances that hinder weight loss and promote fat storage.

One of the most significant ways cortisol sabotages our weight loss goals is by increasing our appetite and cravings for calorie-dense, sugary, and fatty foods. This is due in part to cortisol's effect on our brain's reward system. When we're stressed, our brains crave immediate gratification, and sugary, fatty foods provide a quick burst of pleasure and energy. Additionally, cortisol can interfere with the production of leptin, the hormone that signals to our brain when we're full. This can lead to overeating, even when we're not truly hungry. Furthermore, cortisol promotes the storage of fat, particularly in the abdominal region. This is because cortisol increases the activity of lipoprotein lipase, an enzyme that facilitates fat storage. It also decreases the activity of hormone-sensitive lipase, an enzyme that breaks down stored fat for energy. This shift in enzyme activity favors fat accumulation, particularly around the waistline, leading to the dreaded "stress belly."

The impact of stress on our food choices extends beyond cravings for unhealthy foods. When we're stressed, we're more likely to make impulsive and unhealthy food decisions. We may skip meals, opt for convenience foods, or turn to emotional eating for comfort. These behaviors can further disrupt our metabolism, hinder our weight loss efforts, and contribute to a cycle of stress and unhealthy eating. Stress also affects our gut health, which plays a crucial role in digestion, metabolism, and overall well-being. Studies have shown that stress can alter the composition of our gut microbiome, the trillions of bacteria that reside in our digestive tract. This disruption can lead to inflammation, impaired nutrient absorption, and even weight gain.   The good news is that we can break free from this stress-induced cycle and regain control of our weight and well-being. By understanding the intricate connection between stress and weight gain, we can develop strategies to manage stress, make healthier food choices, and optimize our metabolism.

The first step towards reclaiming your health and achieving your weight loss goals is to understand the intricate ways in which stress can sabotage your efforts. By recognizing the physiological mechanisms at play, you can develop targeted strategies to manage stress and make informed choices that support your metabolism and well-being.

Let's delve deeper into how cortisol, the primary stress hormone, exerts its influence on our bodies. When we encounter a stressful situation, our adrenal glands release cortisol into the bloodstream. This surge of cortisol triggers a series of physiological responses aimed at providing us with the energy and resources to cope with the perceived threat.

One of cortisol's primary functions is to increase blood sugar levels by stimulating the breakdown of glycogen, a stored form of glucose, in the liver. This process, known as gluconeogenesis, ensures that our bodies have a readily available source of energy to fuel the fight-or-flight response. However, when stress becomes chronic, the continuous release of cortisol can lead to chronically elevated blood sugar levels, increasing the risk of insulin resistance and type 2 diabetes.

Furthermore, cortisol promotes the storage of fat, particularly in the abdominal region. This is due in part to cortisol's effect on lipoprotein lipase, an enzyme that facilitates fat storage. When cortisol levels are high, lipoprotein lipase activity increases, leading to increased fat accumulation, particularly around the waistline. This is why chronic stress is often associated with the development of "belly fat" or abdominal obesity.

In addition to its effects on blood sugar and fat storage, cortisol also influences our appetite and cravings. Research has shown that elevated cortisol levels can stimulate appetite and increase our desire for calorie-dense, sugary, and fatty foods. This is due to cortisol's impact on the brain's reward system, which is responsible for our feelings of pleasure and motivation. When we're stressed, our brains crave immediate gratification, and sugary, fatty foods provide a quick burst of pleasure and energy. This can lead to a vicious cycle of stress-induced eating, where we turn to food for comfort, only to experience further weight gain and metabolic disruptions.

Stress also affects our gut health, which plays a crucial role in digestion, metabolism, and overall well-being. The gut microbiome, the trillions of bacteria that reside in our digestive tract, is sensitive to stress. Studies have shown that chronic stress can alter the composition and diversity of our gut microbiome, leading to an imbalance known as dysbiosis. This imbalance can impair nutrient absorption, trigger inflammation, and even contribute to weight gain.

The gut-brain axis, a bidirectional communication system between the gut and the brain, is also affected by stress. When we're stressed, our brains send signals to our gut, which can manifest as digestive problems like bloating, constipation, or diarrhea. Conversely, an unhealthy gut can send signals to the brain, exacerbating stress and anxiety. This vicious cycle further highlights the importance of managing stress for optimal gut health and weight management.

While the effects of stress on our bodies may seem daunting, it's important to remember that we are not powerless. By understanding the science behind the stress-weight connection, we can take proactive steps to mitigate its negative impact.

Incorporating stress-management techniques into our daily routine, such as mindfulness, meditation, yoga, or deep breathing exercises, can help lower cortisol levels and promote relaxation. Engaging in regular exercise, prioritizing sleep, and cultivating a supportive social network can also buffer against the effects of stress.

Additionally, making informed food choices and prioritizing a balanced diet rich in whole, unprocessed foods can help stabilize blood sugar levels, reduce cravings, and nourish our gut microbiome. Green tea, with its calming L-theanine and metabolism-boosting catechins, can be a valuable ally in our stress-management toolkit.

By understanding the intricate relationship between stress and weight gain, we can take charge of our health and create a lifestyle that promotes both physical and mental well-being. The Green Tea Metabolism Makeover is not just about shedding pounds; it's about embracing a holistic approach to health that addresses the mind-body connection and empowers you to live a more balanced, stress-free life.

Mindful Eating: Savoring Your Food and Tuning into Your Body's Signals

I used to be a notorious mindless eater. I would shovel food into my mouth while working, watching TV, or scrolling through my phone, barely registering the taste or texture of what I was consuming. Mealtimes were more of a distraction than a source of nourishment. It wasn't until I discovered the practice of mindful eating that I realized how disconnected I had become from my body's signals and the simple pleasure of savoring a meal.

Mindful eating, a concept rooted in Buddhist philosophy, is about bringing awareness and attention to the present moment during meals. It involves savoring each bite, paying attention to flavors and textures, and tuning into your body's hunger and fullness cues. It's about transforming eating from a mindless act into a mindful experience.

In the context of our Green Tea Metabolism Makeover, mindful eating is a powerful tool that complements the metabolic benefits of green tea. By eating with intention and awareness, we can break free from the cycle of emotional eating, cravings, and mindless snacking that often accompany stress.

When we eat mindfully, we slow down and truly experience our food. We notice the vibrant colors, the enticing aromas, and the subtle nuances of flavor. We chew slowly and deliberately, savoring each bite and allowing our taste buds to fully appreciate the complexity of the meal. By engaging all of our senses, we enhance our enjoyment of food and cultivate a deeper appreciation for the nourishment it provides.   Mindful eating also involves tuning into our body's signals of hunger and fullness. We learn to distinguish between true physical hunger, the gnawing sensation in our stomach that indicates a need for fuel, and emotional hunger, the desire to eat triggered by emotions like stress, boredom, or loneliness. By paying attention to these cues, we can make more conscious choices about when and how much to eat, preventing overeating and promoting a healthier relationship with food.

The benefits of mindful eating extend far beyond weight loss. Research has shown that this practice can reduce stress, improve digestion, enhance nutrient absorption, and promote overall well-being. By focusing on the present moment and fully experiencing our food, we cultivate a sense of gratitude and satisfaction that can transform our relationship with eating and nourish our bodies and minds.

So, how can you incorporate mindful eating into your Green Tea Metabolism Makeover? Here are some practical tips to get you started:

Create a peaceful eating environment: Turn off distractions like the TV, phone, or computer. Sit at a table and focus on your meal.

Engage all your senses: Notice the colors, aromas, flavors, and textures of your food. Take small bites and chew slowly, savoring each mouthful.

Eat slowly: Put down your fork or spoon between bites and take your time. Eating slowly gives your body time to register fullness cues, preventing overeating.

Listen to your body: Pay attention to your hunger and fullness cues. Eat when you're truly hungry and stop when you're comfortably full.

Avoid emotional eating: If you find yourself reaching for food when you're not physically hungry, pause and ask yourself what you're really feeling. Explore alternative ways to cope with your emotions, such as going for a walk, talking to a friend, or practicing deep breathing.

Appreciate your food: Take a moment before eating to appreciate the nourishment that your food provides. Consider the journey it took to get to your plate and the effort involved in its preparation.

Be kind to yourself: Mindful eating is a practice, and it takes time and patience to master. Don't judge yourself if you have moments of mindless eating. Simply acknowledge it and gently bring your attention back to the present moment.

As you delve deeper into mindful eating, you'll discover that it's not just about the mechanics of chewing and tasting. It's about cultivating a sense of gratitude for the nourishment that food provides, acknowledging the interconnectedness of our bodies, minds, and the environment that sustains us. Each meal becomes an opportunity to connect with the present moment, appreciate the flavors and textures of our food, and honor the signals our bodies send us.

By practicing mindful eating, you'll transform your relationship with food from one of mindless consumption to one of conscious nourishment. You'll become more attuned to your body's unique needs and preferences, making food choices that support your health and well-being. You'll also find that you naturally gravitate towards healthier options, as your taste buds become more sensitive and attuned to the subtle nuances of whole, unprocessed foods.

The 28-day Green Tea Metabolism Makeover incorporates mindful eating as a core component, recognizing its transformative power in achieving sustainable weight loss and a healthier lifestyle. By integrating mindful eating practices into your daily routine, you'll enhance the benefits of green tea and create a holistic approach to nourishment that supports your mind, body, and spirit.

Green Tea and Relaxation: Using Green Tea to Reduce Stress

I remember those evenings when stress seemed to wrap around me like a weighted blanket, suffocating my energy and making relaxation feel impossible. In those moments, I would instinctively reach for a cup of tea, the warmth and aroma offering a momentary respite from the chaos. Little did I know that my tea ritual was not merely a comforting habit but a strategic weapon in my arsenal against stress. Green tea, with its unique blend of compounds, holds a secret ingredient that has profound implications for our ability to unwind, de-stress, and ultimately, achieve our weight loss goals.

That secret ingredient is L-theanine, an amino acid found almost exclusively in tea plants. While caffeine is often the star of the show, L-theanine plays a crucial supporting role, working behind the scenes to modulate the effects of caffeine and promote a state of calm alertness. Imagine L-theanine as a gentle hand on your shoulder, guiding you away from the precipice of stress and into a haven of tranquility.

Unlike caffeine, which can sometimes trigger jitters and anxiety, L-theanine has a calming and relaxing effect on the mind and body. It works by increasing the levels of GABA, a neurotransmitter that inhibits overstimulation in the brain, and dopamine, a neurotransmitter associated with pleasure and reward. L-theanine also modulates the levels of serotonin, a neurotransmitter that plays a key role in regulating mood, sleep, and appetite.

This unique combination of effects makes L-theanine a powerful ally in the fight against stress. Studies have shown that L-theanine can reduce anxiety, improve sleep quality, enhance focus and concentration, and even boost mood. It's like a natural tranquilizer, without the drowsiness or side effects of prescription medications.The synergistic relationship between L-theanine and caffeine in green tea is what makes this beverage so effective for stress management. While caffeine provides a gentle energy boost and increased alertness, L-theanine tempers its stimulating effects, preventing the jitters and promoting a state of calm focus. This is why green tea is often described as providing a "calm alertness," a state of mind that is both relaxed and focused, ideal for navigating stressful situations.

In the context of our Green Tea Metabolism Makeover, L-theanine's stress-reducing properties are crucial for achieving our weight loss goals. As we discussed earlier, chronic stress can wreak havoc on our metabolism, leading to increased appetite, cravings, and fat storage. By incorporating green tea into our daily routine, we can harness the power of L-theanine to reduce stress, improve our relationship with food, and optimize our metabolic function.

So, how can you integrate green tea into your stress-management toolkit? Here are a few suggestions:

Create a daily tea ritual: Set aside a few moments each day to savor a cup of green tea. Choose a quiet spot, free from distractions, and allow yourself to fully immerse in the experience. Pay attention to the warmth of the cup in your hands, the aroma that fills your senses, and the delicate flavors that dance on your palate.

Experiment with different varieties: Green tea comes in a wide array of flavors and varieties, each offering a unique experience. Explore different types like matcha, sencha, gyokuro, and genmaicha to find your favorites. You can also try blending green tea with herbs like chamomile, peppermint, or lavender for additional calming effects.

Sip throughout the day: Instead of gulping down a single cup, try sipping on green tea throughout the day. This will help maintain a steady level of L-theanine in your system, promoting sustained relaxation and focus.

Incorporate green tea into your bedtime routine: Enjoy a cup of decaffeinated green tea before bed to promote relaxation and sleep. The calming effects of L-theanine can help you unwind from the day's stresses and prepare for a restful night's sleep.

Pair green tea with stress-reducing activities: Combine your tea ritual with other stress-management techniques, such as deep breathing exercises, meditation, or gentle yoga. This can create a powerful synergistic effect, amplifying the relaxation response and enhancing your overall well-being.

Get creative with green tea: Don't limit yourself to just drinking green tea. Explore other ways to incorporate it into your routine, such as adding matcha powder to smoothies or yogurt, using green tea bags in a bath, or trying green tea-infused skincare products.

As you experiment with different ways to incorporate green tea into your life, you'll discover that it's not just a beverage; it's a versatile tool for stress management, relaxation, and overall well-being. Whether you're enjoying a cup of matcha during a midday break, sipping on sencha while working, or unwinding with a chamomile green tea blend before bed, each sip is an opportunity to invite tranquility into your life and support your journey towards a healthier, happier you.

While scientific research continues to uncover the full potential of L-theanine, one thing is clear: this remarkable amino acid holds the key to unlocking a calmer, more focused, and less stressed version of ourselves. By harnessing the power of L-theanine in green tea, we can break free from the grip of stress and embrace a more balanced and fulfilling life.

As you progress through your Green Tea Metabolism Makeover, remember that managing stress is not just about shedding pounds; it's about cultivating a deeper connection with your mind and body. By integrating stress-reducing practices like mindful eating, regular exercise, and green tea consumption into your daily routine, you'll create a powerful synergy that promotes overall well-being, enhances your metabolism, and paves the way for sustainable weight loss.

So, the next time you feel stress creeping in, reach for a cup of green tea. Let the warmth of the cup soothe your soul, the aroma awaken your senses, and the delicate flavors transport you to a state of tranquility. With each sip, you're not just enjoying a delicious beverage; you're nurturing your mind and body, creating a haven of calm amidst the chaos of daily life.

Remember, your journey towards a healthier, happier you is not just about the destination; it's about the path you take to get there. Embrace the power of green tea and allow its calming embrace to guide you on your path to stress-free living and sustainable weight loss.

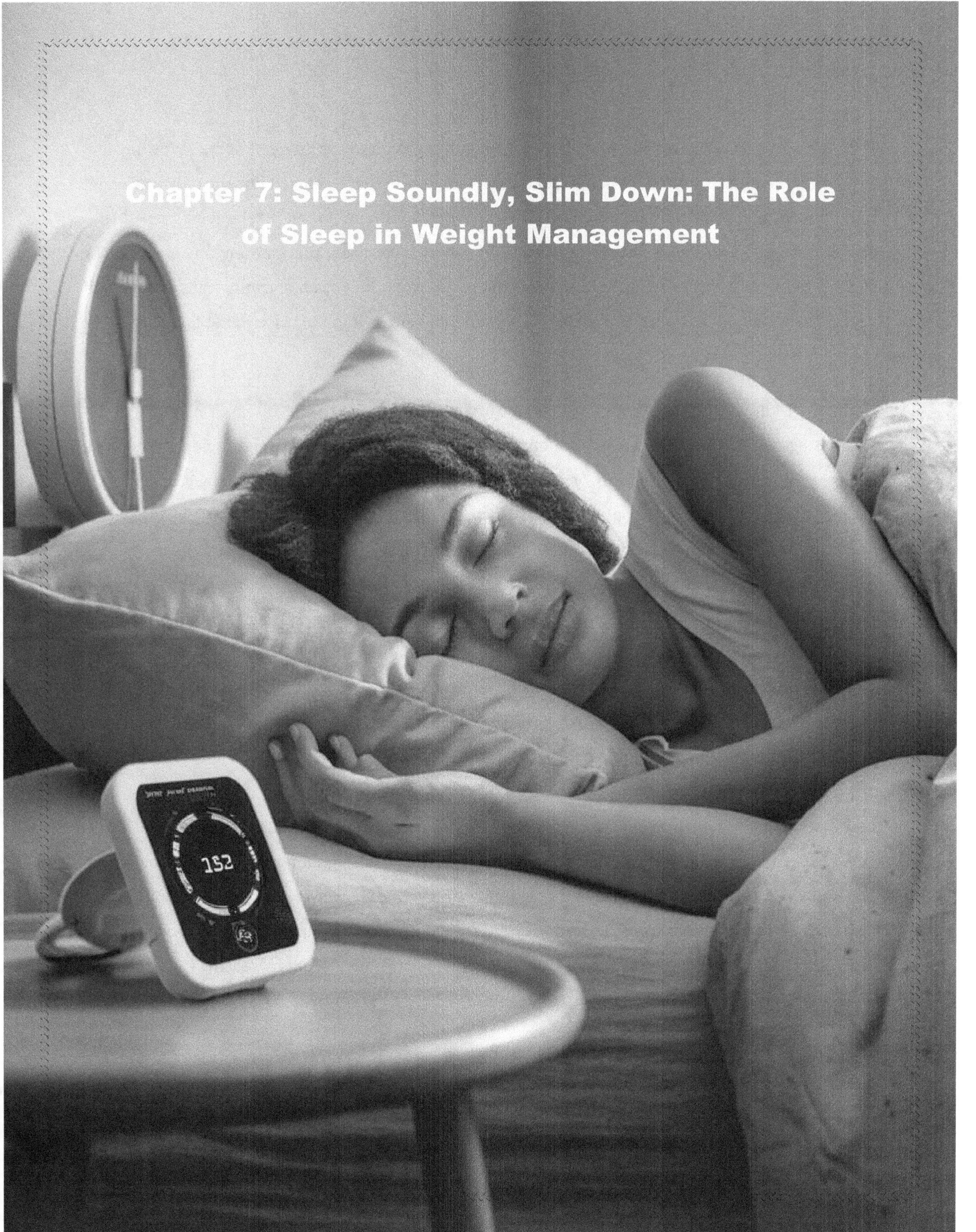
Chapter 7: Sleep Soundly, Slim Down: The Role of Sleep in Weight Management

There was a time in my life when burning the midnight oil was a badge of honor. Working late into the night, fueled by caffeine and the thrill of productivity, seemed like the only way to get ahead. Sleep was a luxury I could ill afford, or so I thought. But as the days turned into sleepless nights, I noticed a disturbing trend. My energy levels were plummeting, my cravings for sugary treats were skyrocketing, and my waistline was expanding at an alarming rate. It was as if my body was rebelling against my neglect of sleep, and I was paying the price in the form of weight gain and fatigue.

Little did I know that my experience was not unique. In fact, scientific research has unveiled a fascinating and complex connection between sleep deprivation and weight gain. When we consistently shortchange ourselves on sleep, we disrupt a delicate hormonal balance that plays a crucial role in regulating our appetite, metabolism, and body composition. Two key players in this hormonal orchestra are ghrelin and leptin. Ghrelin, often dubbed the "hunger hormone," is produced in the stomach and signals to the brain when it's time to eat. When we're well-rested, ghrelin levels rise before meals and decrease after we've eaten, helping us maintain a healthy appetite and energy balance. However, when we're sleep-deprived, ghrelin levels remain elevated, sending constant hunger signals to our brains and increasing our desire to eat. This can lead to overeating, particularly of calorie-dense, sugary, and fatty foods, which provide a quick energy boost but ultimately contribute to weight gain.

Leptin, on the other hand, is the "satiety hormone" that tells our brains when we're full and should stop eating. When we're well-rested, leptin levels rise after meals, signaling to our brains that we've had enough and promoting a sense of fullness and satisfaction. However, sleep deprivation throws a wrench into this system, causing leptin levels to decrease. This means our brains receive fewer signals of fullness, making it harder for us to feel satisfied after meals and increasing the likelihood of overeating.

The combined effect of increased ghrelin and decreased leptin is a recipe for disaster when it comes to weight management. We feel hungrier, crave more unhealthy foods, and find it harder to stop eating even when we're full. This hormonal imbalance creates a perfect storm for weight gain, especially when combined with the other metabolic disruptions caused by sleep deprivation.

Sleep deprivation not only disrupts our hunger and satiety hormones but also impairs our glucose metabolism. When we don't get enough sleep, our bodies become less efficient at utilizing glucose, the sugar that fuels our cells. This can lead to elevated blood sugar levels, insulin resistance, and ultimately, increased fat storage. Insulin, a hormone that helps regulate blood sugar, becomes less effective at its job, forcing the pancreas to produce more insulin to compensate. Over time, this can lead to insulin resistance, a condition in which cells become less responsive to insulin's signals, increasing the risk of type 2 diabetes and other metabolic disorders.   In addition to its impact on glucose metabolism, sleep deprivation also affects our energy expenditure, the number of calories we burn throughout the day. When we're sleep-deprived, we tend to be less active and more sedentary, leading to a decrease in energy expenditure. Furthermore, studies have shown that sleep deprivation can lower our resting metabolic rate (RMR), the number of calories our bodies burn at rest. This means that even when we're not moving, we're burning fewer calories, further contributing to weight gain.

The link between sleep deprivation and weight gain is not just theoretical; numerous studies have confirmed this association. Research has consistently shown that individuals who sleep less than seven hours per night are more likely to be overweight or obese compared to those who get adequate sleep. In fact, some studies have suggested that each hour of sleep lost per night is associated with a 0.35 kg/m2 increase in body mass index (BMI).

A landmark study published in the journal SLEEP followed over 68,000 women for 16 years and found that those who slept five hours or less per night were 15% more likely to become obese than those who slept seven hours. Another study published in the American Journal of Clinical Nutrition found that short sleep duration was associated with increased abdominal fat, even after adjusting for other factors like diet and physical activity.

The evidence is clear: sleep deprivation is a significant risk factor for weight gain and obesity. But why is this the case? Researchers believe that the hormonal imbalances and metabolic disruptions caused by lack of sleep create a perfect storm for weight gain.

When we're sleep-deprived, our bodies crave calorie-dense, sugary, and fatty foods to compensate for the lack of energy and to provide a quick dopamine hit to the brain's reward system. At the same time, our bodies become less efficient at utilizing glucose and burning calories, leading to increased fat storage. This combination of increased calorie intake and decreased calorie expenditure creates a recipe for weight gain.

Furthermore, sleep deprivation can also affect our decision-making abilities, making us more likely to choose unhealthy foods and less likely to engage in physical activity. When we're tired and stressed, we're less likely to make rational choices about what we eat and more likely to succumb to cravings for comfort foods. We're also less likely to have the energy or motivation to exercise, further exacerbating the problem.

The good news is that we have the power to break this cycle and reclaim our sleep, our health, and our weight. By prioritizing sleep and adopting healthy sleep habits, we can restore hormonal balance, optimize metabolism, and create a more conducive environment for weight loss. This means aiming for 7-8 hours of sleep per night, establishing a consistent sleep schedule, creating a relaxing bedtime routine, and optimizing our sleep environment.

Incorporating green tea into your daily routine can also be beneficial for improving sleep quality. The L-theanine in green tea promotes relaxation and reduces anxiety, making it easier to fall asleep and stay asleep. Consider enjoying a cup of decaffeinated green tea before bed to reap these benefits without the stimulating effects of caffeine.

Remember, sleep is not a luxury; it's a necessity for optimal health and well-being. By prioritizing sleep and adopting a healthy lifestyle, you can break free from the grip of sleep deprivation, improve your metabolism, and achieve your weight loss goals.

Creating a Sleep Sanctuary: Tips for a Restful Night's Sleep

Transforming your sleep into a rejuvenating experience is a cornerstone of the Green Tea Metabolism Makeover. As we've explored, quality sleep isn't merely about feeling rested; it's a metabolic powerhouse, influencing your hormones, appetite, and energy levels. Creating a sleep sanctuary – a tranquil oasis where your body can rest and repair – is essential for unlocking your full fat-burning potential and achieving lasting weight loss.Imagine stepping into a haven of serenity each night, a space designed to promote deep relaxation and restorative slumber. Your sleep sanctuary is more than just a bedroom; it's a carefully curated environment that caters to your body's natural sleep rhythms and encourages optimal rest. By implementing a few simple yet effective strategies, you can transform your sleep into a rejuvenating ritual that leaves you feeling refreshed, revitalized, and ready to conquer your day.

One of the most fundamental pillars of healthy sleep is establishing a consistent sleep schedule. Our bodies thrive on routine, and our internal clocks, known as circadian rhythms, dictate our natural sleep-wake cycles. By going to bed and waking up at the same time each day, even on weekends, we can reinforce these rhythms and promote more restful sleep.

Think of your sleep schedule as a rhythmic dance between light and darkness, activity and rest. As daylight fades, our bodies begin to produce melatonin, a hormone that signals it's time to unwind and prepare for sleep. Conversely, as the sun rises, our bodies naturally suppress melatonin and increase cortisol production, promoting wakefulness and alertness. By adhering to a consistent sleep schedule, we align ourselves with these natural rhythms, making it easier to fall asleep and wake up feeling refreshed.

Creating a tranquil sleep environment is equally important. Imagine your bedroom as a cozy cocoon, shielded from the distractions and disturbances of the outside world. Dim the lights, draw the curtains, and create a serene atmosphere that invites relaxation and sleep. Consider using blackout curtains or an eye mask to block out any unwanted light, as even a small amount of light can disrupt melatonin production and interfere with sleep.

Noise can also be a major sleep disruptor. If your bedroom is prone to noise from traffic, neighbors, or other sources, consider using earplugs or a white noise machine to create a peaceful soundscape. You can also try playing calming music or nature sounds to mask unwanted noise and promote relaxation.

The temperature of your bedroom can also impact your sleep quality. Most experts recommend keeping your bedroom cool, ideally between 60 and 67 degrees Fahrenheit. A cool room temperature helps lower your body's core temperature, which is a natural signal for sleep. You can achieve this by adjusting your thermostat, using a fan, or opting for lighter bedding. As bedtime approaches, it's important to avoid substances that can interfere with sleep. Caffeine, a stimulant found in coffee, tea, chocolate, and some medications, can disrupt your sleep-wake cycle and make it harder to fall asleep. Aim to avoid caffeine for at least six hours before bed to allow your body to wind down naturally.

Electronics, such as smartphones, tablets, and computers, emit blue light that can suppress melatonin production and interfere with sleep. The blue light tricks our brains into thinking it's still daytime, making it difficult to relax and fall asleep. Make it a habit to disconnect from electronics at least an hour before bed and opt for relaxing activities like reading, taking a bath, or meditating. Finally, managing stress is crucial for achieving restful sleep. Stress triggers the release of cortisol, a hormone that can interfere with sleep and contribute to weight gain. Incorporate stress-management techniques into your daily routine, such as mindfulness, meditation, deep breathing exercises, or yoga. These practices can help calm your mind and body, reduce cortisol levels, and prepare you for a peaceful night's sleep.

Remember, creating a sleep sanctuary is a personal journey. Experiment with different strategies and find what works best for you. By prioritizing sleep and creating a restful environment, you'll not only improve your sleep quality but also enhance your metabolism, reduce stress, and achieve your weight loss goals.

Chapter 8

Hydration for Health: The Importance of Water in Weight Loss

"Water is the driving force of all nature." - Leonardo da Vinci

Leonardo da Vinci's words resonate deeply when we consider the profound impact of water on our bodies and overall health. It's easy to overlook this humble liquid, yet it's the most abundant substance in our bodies, comprising roughly 60% of our total weight. Every cell, tissue, and organ depends on water to function properly. It's the lifeblood that courses through our veins, transporting nutrients, oxygen, and waste products throughout our system.

In the grand symphony of bodily functions, water plays a starring role in the intricate dance of digestion. As we consume food, water helps break it down, facilitating the absorption of essential nutrients and the elimination of waste products. It acts as a lubricant, ensuring smooth movement throughout the digestive tract, preventing constipation and promoting regularity. Adequate hydration is crucial for maintaining a healthy gut microbiome, the trillions of bacteria that reside in our digestive system and play a vital role in our overall health and well-being.

Beyond digestion, water is a key player in our metabolic processes, the intricate chemical reactions that convert food into energy. Every metabolic pathway, from the breakdown of carbohydrates and fats to the synthesis of proteins and enzymes, relies on water as a medium. When we're dehydrated, these processes slow down, hindering our metabolism and making it harder to burn calories and lose weight.

Think of your metabolism as a well-oiled machine, with water acting as the lubricant that keeps everything running smoothly. When you're well-hydrated, your metabolic engine hums along efficiently, burning calories and utilizing nutrients effectively. But when you're dehydrated, the machine sputters and slows down, making it more difficult to achieve your weight loss goals.

Water also plays a crucial role in temperature regulation, keeping our bodies cool and preventing overheating during exercise or hot weather. As we sweat, water evaporates from our skin, taking heat with it and lowering our body temperature. Without adequate hydration, our bodies struggle to regulate temperature, leading to heat exhaustion, heat stroke, and other heat-related illnesses. By staying hydrated, we ensure our bodies can effectively cool themselves down, allowing us to exercise longer and harder, ultimately burning more calories and accelerating our weight loss journey.

In addition to its roles in digestion, metabolism, and temperature regulation, water is also essential for detoxification, the process by which our bodies eliminate waste products and toxins. Our kidneys, the primary organs responsible for filtering waste from the blood, rely on water to function properly. When we're dehydrated, our kidneys have to work harder to remove waste, which can put a strain on these vital organs and lead to a buildup of toxins in our system. By staying hydrated, we support our kidneys' detoxification efforts, promoting overall health and well-being.

Now, let's explore how adequate hydration can specifically support your weight loss goals. One of the most significant ways water aids in weight loss is by promoting satiety, the feeling of fullness and satisfaction after a meal. When we drink water before or during a meal, it fills up our stomachs, reducing the amount of food we consume. This can lead to a lower calorie intake and contribute to gradual weight loss over time.

Moreover, research suggests that drinking water may temporarily increase our metabolic rate, the number of calories our bodies burn at rest. While the exact mechanism is still under investigation, studies have shown that drinking cold water can boost metabolism by up to 30% for a short period. This is likely due to the energy required to warm the water to body temperature, a process known as thermogenesis.

Staying hydrated can also improve our exercise performance and endurance. When we're dehydrated, our blood volume decreases, making it harder for our hearts to pump blood and deliver oxygen to our muscles. This can lead to fatigue, cramping, and decreased exercise performance. By drinking plenty of water before, during, and after exercise, we can maintain optimal hydration levels, allowing us to push harder and longer, burning more calories in the process.

Incorporating green tea into your hydration routine can further enhance the benefits of water. Green tea not only provides additional fluids but also delivers a dose of antioxidants and metabolism-boosting compounds like catechins and EGCG. These compounds can work synergistically with water to increase fat oxidation, improve insulin sensitivity, and reduce inflammation, all of which contribute to weight loss and overall health.

Water: The Essential Nutrient for Weight Loss and Overall Health

"Thousands have lived without love, not one without water." - W.H. Auden

In the quest for optimal health and a successful metabolism makeover, we often focus on intricate dietary plans and rigorous exercise regimens. However, amidst the complexities of nutrition and fitness, there lies a simple yet powerful element that is often overlooked: water. Often underestimated, water is far more than just a thirst quencher. It's the lifeblood that courses through our veins, the unsung hero that fuels every cell, tissue, and organ, and the key to unlocking our body's full potential.

Imagine your body as a bustling metropolis, a complex network of systems working together to sustain life. Water is the infrastructure that keeps this city running smoothly. It's the transportation system that delivers nutrients and oxygen to every corner, the sanitation department that removes waste products, and the climate control system that regulates temperature. Without adequate water, this intricate city grinds to a halt, its functions compromised, and its inhabitants struggling to thrive.

Let's delve into the multifaceted roles water plays in our bodies, starting with digestion. As we consume food, water helps break it down into smaller particles, facilitating the absorption of essential nutrients and the elimination of waste products. It acts as a lubricant, ensuring smooth movement throughout the digestive tract and preventing constipation. A well-hydrated digestive system is key to optimal nutrient absorption and a healthy gut microbiome, the trillions of bacteria that reside in our intestines and play a vital role in our overall health and well-being.

Beyond digestion, water is a key player in our metabolic processes, the intricate chemical reactions that convert food into energy. Every metabolic pathway, from the breakdown of carbohydrates and fats to the synthesis of proteins and enzymes, relies on water as a medium. When we're dehydrated, these processes slow down, hindering our metabolism and making it harder to burn calories and lose weight.

Think of your metabolism as a well-oiled machine, with water acting as the lubricant that keeps everything running smoothly. When you're well-hydrated, your metabolic engine hums along efficiently, burning calories and utilizing nutrients effectively. But when you're dehydrated, the machine sputters and slows down, making it more difficult to achieve your weight loss goals. Water also plays a crucial role in temperature regulation, keeping our bodies cool and preventing overheating during exercise or hot weather. As we sweat, water evaporates from our skin, taking heat with it and lowering our body temperature. Without adequate hydration, our bodies struggle to regulate temperature, leading to heat exhaustion, heat stroke, and other heat-related illnesses. By staying hydrated, we ensure our bodies can effectively cool themselves down, allowing us to exercise longer and harder, ultimately burning more calories and accelerating our weight loss journey.

In addition to its roles in digestion, metabolism, and temperature regulation, water is also essential for detoxification, the process by which our bodies eliminate waste products and toxins. Our kidneys, the primary organs responsible for filtering waste from the blood, rely on water to function properly. When we're dehydrated, our kidneys have to work harder to remove waste, which can put a strain on these vital organs and lead to a buildup of toxins in our system. By staying hydrated, we support our kidneys' detoxification efforts, promoting overall health and well-being.

Now, let's explore how adequate hydration can specifically support your weight loss goals. One of the most significant ways water aids in weight loss is by promoting satiety, the feeling of fullness and satisfaction after a meal. When we drink water before or during a meal, it fills up our stomachs, reducing the amount of food we consume. This can lead to a lower calorie intake and contribute to gradual weight loss over time. Studies have shown that individuals who drink water before meals tend to consume fewer calories and lose more weight compared to those who don't. Moreover, research suggests that drinking water may temporarily increase our metabolic rate, the number of calories our bodies burn at rest. While the exact mechanism is still under investigation, studies have shown that drinking cold water can boost metabolism by up to 30% for a short period. This is likely due to the energy required to warm the water to body temperature, a process known as thermogenesis.

Staying hydrated can also improve our exercise performance and endurance. When we're dehydrated, our blood volume decreases, making it harder for our hearts to pump blood and deliver oxygen to our muscles. This can lead to fatigue, cramping, and decreased exercise performance. By drinking plenty of water before, during, and after exercise, we can maintain optimal hydration levels, allowing us to push harder and longer, burning more calories in the process.

Incorporating green tea into your hydration routine can further enhance the benefits of water. Green tea not only provides additional fluids but also delivers a dose of antioxidants and metabolism-boosting compounds like catechins and EGCG. These compounds can work synergistically with water to increase fat oxidation, improve insulin sensitivity, and reduce inflammation, all of which contribute to weight loss and overall health.

Green Tea and Hydration: How Green Tea Can Contribute to Your Daily Fluid Intake

Let's address a common myth that might be hindering your hydration journey: the belief that caffeinated beverages, like green tea, are dehydrating. This misconception has lingered for years, casting a shadow of doubt on the hydrating potential of this beloved beverage. However, scientific evidence paints a different picture, revealing that green tea can, in fact, contribute to your daily fluid intake and support your overall hydration goals.

It's true that caffeine, a natural stimulant found in green tea, has a mild diuretic effect. This means it can temporarily increase urine production, leading to the perception that it might dehydrate you. However, numerous studies have shown that the diuretic effect of caffeine is minimal when consumed in moderate amounts, as typically found in a few cups of green tea.In fact, research has demonstrated that caffeinated beverages like green tea can be just as hydrating as plain water. The fluid you consume from green tea outweighs any potential diuretic effect, contributing to your overall fluid balance and supporting your hydration needs.

So, how does green tea contribute to hydration? Firstly, it's primarily composed of water, just like any other beverage. Each cup of green tea you enjoy adds to your daily fluid intake, helping you meet your hydration goals. But green tea goes beyond simple hydration. It's a rich source of antioxidants, including catechins like EGCG, which have been linked to numerous health benefits, including improved metabolism and fat burning. These antioxidants can help protect your cells from damage caused by free radicals, unstable molecules that can contribute to inflammation and chronic diseases.Furthermore, green tea contains electrolytes, essential minerals that help maintain fluid balance in your body. Sodium, potassium, and magnesium, all found in green tea, play a vital role in regulating hydration levels and ensuring proper muscle and nerve function.

While green tea can be a valuable addition to your hydration routine, it's important to be mindful of its caffeine content. Excessive caffeine intake can lead to side effects like jitters, anxiety, and sleep disturbances. Therefore, it's best to limit your consumption to 3-4 cups of green tea per day, especially if you're sensitive to caffeine. If you're concerned about caffeine, opt for decaffeinated green tea, which still offers the hydrating benefits and antioxidants without the stimulating effects of caffeine. You can also enjoy green tea alongside plain water throughout the day, ensuring you're getting a variety of fluids and maximizing your hydration potential.

Incorporating green tea into your 28-day Green Tea Metabolism Makeover can be a delicious and effective way to support your hydration goals. Start your day with a revitalizing matcha latte, enjoy a refreshing cup of sencha during your workday, or unwind with a calming cup of chamomile green tea before bed. Beyond its hydrating properties, green tea offers a wealth of additional benefits that can enhance your overall health and well-being. Its antioxidants may protect against chronic diseases, its metabolism-boosting compounds can aid in weight loss, and its calming L-theanine can promote relaxation and reduce stress. By embracing green tea as a part of your daily routine, you're not only quenching your thirst but also nourishing your body from the inside out.

So, let go of the misconception that caffeinated beverages are dehydrating and embrace the hydrating power of green tea. With its refreshing taste, abundance of antioxidants, and potential metabolic benefits, green tea is a valuable addition to your hydration arsenal, supporting your weight loss journey and promoting overall health and vitality.

Flavorful Water Infusions: Adding a Twist to Your Hydration Routine

In the quest for optimal health and a revitalized metabolism, water is our unsung hero. But let's face it, plain water, while essential, can sometimes feel a bit lackluster. Fear not! We're about to embark on a flavor-filled adventure, transforming your hydration routine into a delightful symphony of taste and well-being. By infusing your water with the invigorating essence of green tea and a medley of fruits, herbs, and spices, you'll create refreshing elixirs that not only quench your thirst but also tantalize your taste buds and support your weight loss goals. Imagine a pitcher filled with crystal-clear water, adorned with vibrant slices of citrus fruits, fragrant sprigs of mint, and delicate cucumber ribbons. As these ingredients mingle and infuse, they release their aromatic oils and subtle flavors, transforming ordinary water into a spa-like experience. And at the heart of this transformation lies green tea, its subtle earthiness and antioxidant power adding a unique dimension to each sip.

Green tea, with its metabolism-boosting catechins and calming L-theanine, is the perfect base for creating flavorful water infusions. Its gentle taste complements a variety of fruits, herbs, and spices, allowing you to customize your hydration experience to your liking. Whether you prefer a citrusy burst, a hint of mint, or a touch of spice, the possibilities are endless.

To embark on this flavor adventure, let's explore a few enticing green tea-infused water combinations that will leave you feeling refreshed, revitalized, and ready to conquer your day.

Citrus Symphony: Combine slices of lemon, lime, and orange with a few sprigs of fresh mint and a green tea bag. Let it steep in the refrigerator for a few hours, allowing the flavors to meld and create a refreshing citrus symphony. The combination of zesty citrus, cool mint, and the subtle earthiness of green tea is a delightful way to start your day or re-energize in the afternoon.

Berry Bliss: Muddle a handful of fresh or frozen berries (strawberries, raspberries, blueberries) in a pitcher. Add a few slices of cucumber for a touch of coolness and a green tea bag. Let it infuse overnight in the refrigerator for a vibrant and antioxidant-rich beverage. The sweetness of the berries, the subtle cucumber notes, and the earthiness of green tea create a harmonious blend that will tantalize your taste buds and leave you feeling refreshed.

Tropical Paradise: Transport yourself to a tropical paradise with this exotic infusion. Combine chunks of pineapple, mango, and a few slices of ginger with a green tea bag. Let it steep in the refrigerator for a few hours, allowing the flavors to meld and create a taste of the tropics. The sweetness of the fruits, the subtle heat of the ginger, and the earthy notes of green tea will transport you to a sunny beach, even if you're stuck at your desk.

Herbal Harmony: For a more calming and soothing experience, try combining green tea with chamomile flowers, lavender buds, and a few slices of lemon. Let it steep in the refrigerator overnight for a relaxing and aromatic infusion. The floral notes of chamomile and lavender, combined with the citrusy brightness of lemon and the subtle earthiness of green tea, create a harmonious blend that promotes relaxation and tranquility.

Spicy Sensation: Add a touch of spice to your hydration routine with this invigorating infusion. Combine slices of cucumber, jalapeño peppers (seeds removed for less heat), and a green tea bag. Let it steep in the refrigerator for a few hours, allowing the flavors to meld and create a refreshing and spicy sensation. The coolness of the cucumber, the subtle heat of the jalapeño, and the earthiness of green tea will awaken your senses and leave you feeling energized.

These are just a few ideas to ignite your creativity and inspire you to experiment with your own unique flavor combinations. Feel free to mix and match different fruits, herbs, and spices to create your signature green tea-infused water. The possibilities are endless, and the journey of discovery is part of the fun!

As you embark on this flavor-filled adventure, remember a few key tips to ensure your green tea infusions are both delicious and beneficial:

Use high-quality ingredients: Opt for fresh, organic fruits, herbs, and spices whenever possible. Their vibrant flavors and aromas will elevate your water infusions to a whole new level.

Experiment with different green tea varieties: Each type of green tea offers a unique flavor profile. Try using matcha, sencha, gyokuro, or other varieties to create diverse and exciting infusions.

Adjust steeping time to your preference: The longer you steep your infusion, the stronger the flavor will be. Start with a shorter steeping time and gradually increase it until you find the perfect balance for your taste buds.

Serve chilled: Green tea-infused water is most refreshing when served cold. Prepare a large batch in the morning and keep it in the refrigerator throughout the day for a readily available hydration boost.

Get creative with presentation: Add a touch of elegance to your water infusions by serving them in mason jars, glass pitchers, or wine glasses. Garnish with fresh herbs, fruit slices, or edible flowers for a visually appealing and enticing drink.

By incorporating green tea-infused water into your daily routine, you'll not only enhance your hydration but also nourish your body with antioxidants and metabolism-boosting compounds. So, let your creativity flow and discover the endless possibilities of flavorful water infusions. With each sip, you'll be one step closer to achieving your Green Tea Metabolism Makeover goals and embracing a healthier, more vibrant you.

Chapter 9: Gut Feeling: The Microbiome's Role in Metabolism and Weight

"All disease begins in the gut." - Hippocrates

The ancient Greek physician Hippocrates, often considered the father of medicine, recognized a profound truth over two millennia ago: the gut plays a pivotal role in our overall health and well-being. While his words may have seemed intuitive at the time, modern science is now revealing the intricate mechanisms behind this connection, uncovering a hidden world within our digestive system that holds the key to unlocking a healthier, leaner, and more vibrant you.

Welcome to the fascinating world of the gut microbiome, a bustling metropolis of trillions of microorganisms residing within our digestive tract. This microscopic community, comprised of bacteria, viruses, fungi, and other microbes, plays a far more significant role in our health than we ever imagined. In fact, scientists now believe that the gut microbiome may be as influential as our own genes in determining our susceptibility to various diseases, including obesity, diabetes, heart disease, and even mental health disorders.

Think of your gut microbiome as a complex ecosystem, teeming with diverse life forms that interact with each other and with your body in a delicate balance. When this balance is disrupted, known as dysbiosis, it can trigger a cascade of negative effects, impacting everything from digestion and nutrient absorption to immune function and metabolism. And as we'll explore in this chapter, an imbalanced gut microbiome can significantly hinder your weight loss efforts and contribute to metabolic dysfunction.

The gut-weight connection is a fascinating and complex interplay of factors. Research suggests that the composition of our gut microbiome can influence how efficiently we extract energy from food, how we store fat, and even how our bodies regulate appetite and satiety signals. Certain types of gut bacteria are more efficient at extracting calories from food, while others promote fat storage and inflammation. An imbalance in these bacterial populations can tip the scales in favor of weight gain and metabolic dysfunction.

Furthermore, the gut microbiome plays a crucial role in regulating our immune system and inflammatory responses. When the balance of gut bacteria is disrupted, it can lead to chronic low-grade inflammation, which has been linked to obesity, insulin resistance, and other metabolic disorders. An imbalanced gut microbiome can also impair the integrity of the gut barrier, allowing harmful substances to leak into the bloodstream and trigger further inflammation throughout the body.So, how can we nurture a healthy gut microbiome and support our weight loss goals? The answer lies in a combination of dietary and lifestyle choices that promote a diverse and balanced gut ecosystem.

One of the most effective ways to foster a healthy gut is by consuming a diet rich in fiber. Fiber acts as a prebiotic, providing nourishment for the beneficial bacteria in our gut. These bacteria, in turn, produce short-chain fatty acids, which have been shown to improve metabolism, reduce inflammation, and promote satiety. Aim to include plenty of fiber-rich foods in your diet, such as fruits, vegetables, whole grains, and legumes.

Probiotics, live microorganisms that confer health benefits when consumed in adequate amounts, can also play a role in promoting a healthy gut microbiome. Foods like yogurt, kefir, sauerkraut, and kimchi are rich in probiotics and can help replenish and diversify the bacterial populations in your gut. Consider incorporating these fermented foods into your diet regularly to support your gut health and overall well-being.

In addition to fiber and probiotics, certain polyphenols found in plant foods, including green tea, may also have prebiotic effects, promoting the growth of beneficial gut bacteria. Emerging research suggests that green tea's catechins, particularly EGCG, may selectively inhibit the growth of harmful bacteria while fostering the growth of beneficial bacteria. This could potentially contribute to a more balanced gut microbiome and support weight loss efforts.

While the exact mechanisms through which green tea influences the gut microbiome are still under investigation, studies have shown promising results. One study published in the Journal of Nutritional Biochemistry found that green tea extract supplementation led to a significant increase in beneficial bacteria and a decrease in harmful bacteria in the gut of obese mice. Another study in the European Journal of Nutrition showed that green tea consumption was associated with a more diverse gut microbiome in humans.

The potential prebiotic effects of green tea add another layer to its already impressive list of health benefits. By promoting a healthy gut microbiome, green tea can help optimize digestion, nutrient absorption, immune function, and metabolism, all of which play a crucial role in achieving and maintaining a healthy weight.

The Gut-Weight Connection: How Your Gut Bacteria Can Influence Your Weight

Deep within your digestive system, an intricate world teeming with trillions of microorganisms thrives—a bustling metropolis of bacteria, viruses, fungi, and other microbes collectively known as the gut microbiome. This hidden universe, once largely overlooked, is now recognized as a key player in our overall health, influencing everything from digestion and nutrient absorption to immune function and even our metabolism. It's a fascinating ecosystem where balance is key, and disruptions can have far-reaching consequences, including impacting your weight loss journey.

Imagine your gut microbiome as a vibrant rainforest, teeming with diverse life forms, each playing a unique role in maintaining the delicate balance of this ecosystem. When this balance is disrupted, known as dysbiosis, it's like a wildfire sweeping through the rainforest, leaving destruction in its wake. This imbalance can trigger a cascade of negative effects, impacting your metabolism and potentially hindering your efforts to achieve a healthy weight.

The gut-weight connection is a complex and fascinating interplay of factors, where the composition of your gut microbiome can significantly influence how your body processes food, extracts energy, and stores fat. Certain types of gut bacteria are more adept at extracting calories from the food you eat, while others play a role in fat storage and inflammation. An imbalance in these bacterial populations can tip the scales in favor of weight gain and metabolic dysfunction.

Think of your gut microbiome as a team of metabolic managers, each with a specific role in processing the food you consume. Some bacteria are like efficient energy harvesters, extracting every last calorie from your food, while others are more like thrifty savers, promoting fat storage for future use. When the balance tips towards the energy harvesters, you may find it easier to gain weight, even if you're eating a healthy diet. Conversely, a microbiome dominated by bacteria that promote fat storage can make weight loss more challenging, as your body becomes more efficient at holding onto those extra calories.

But the gut microbiome's influence on weight goes beyond just calorie extraction and fat storage. It also plays a crucial role in regulating your appetite and satiety signals. Certain gut bacteria produce hormones that communicate with your brain, influencing your feelings of hunger and fullness.

An imbalance in these bacteria can disrupt these signals, leading to increased appetite, cravings, and overeating. It's like having a team of misinformed advisors sending conflicting messages to your brain, making it difficult to listen to your body's true hunger cues.

Furthermore, the gut microbiome plays a vital role in regulating inflammation, a key factor in metabolic health and weight management. When the balance of gut bacteria is disrupted, it can lead to chronic low-grade inflammation throughout the body. This inflammation can interfere with insulin signaling, making it harder for your body to use glucose for energy and increasing the risk of insulin resistance, a major contributor to metabolic syndrome and type 2 diabetes. Chronic inflammation can also promote fat storage and hinder your body's ability to burn fat effectively.

The gut-weight connection is a dynamic and ongoing interplay between your microbiome and your metabolism. By understanding this connection, you can take proactive steps to nurture a healthy gut microbiome and support your weight loss goals. Incorporating green tea into your daily routine is one such step. Green tea, with its rich array of antioxidants and polyphenols, has been shown to have prebiotic effects, promoting the growth of beneficial gut bacteria.

Emerging research suggests that green tea's catechins, particularly EGCG, may selectively inhibit the growth of harmful bacteria while fostering the growth of beneficial bacteria. This could potentially lead to a more balanced gut microbiome, supporting healthy metabolism and weight management. While more research is needed to fully understand the mechanisms behind green tea's impact on the gut microbiome, the existing evidence suggests a promising connection.

As you embark on your Green Tea Metabolism Makeover, remember that your gut microbiome is a powerful ally in your journey towards a healthier, leaner you. By nourishing your gut with a balanced diet rich in fiber, probiotics, and green tea, you'll be cultivating a thriving ecosystem that supports optimal metabolism, reduces inflammation, and helps you achieve your weight loss goals.

Feeding Your Friendly Bacteria: Probiotic and Prebiotic Foods for a Healthy Gut

Within the depths of your gut lies a bustling metropolis, a complex ecosystem teeming with trillions of microorganisms known as the gut microbiome. This microbial community plays a crucial role in your overall health, influencing everything from digestion and nutrient absorption to immune function and metabolism. Like a well-tended garden, your gut microbiome requires careful nurturing to flourish and support your weight loss goals.

In this chapter, we'll delve into the fascinating world of probiotics and prebiotics, the dynamic duo that can help cultivate a healthy gut ecosystem and optimize your metabolic function.

Think of probiotics as the "good guys" of your gut, the beneficial bacteria that contribute to a balanced and thriving microbiome. These live microorganisms, when consumed in adequate amounts, confer a host of health benefits, including improved digestion, enhanced immune function, and even potential weight management support. They work by competing with harmful bacteria for space and resources, producing beneficial compounds like short-chain fatty acids, and interacting with your immune system to promote a healthy inflammatory response.

Probiotic-rich foods are like tiny capsules of beneficial bacteria, ready to colonize your gut and restore balance to your microbiome. Yogurt, a creamy and versatile dairy product, is a classic source of probiotics, particularly those containing live and active cultures. Look for yogurts with strains like Lactobacillus and Bifidobacterium, which have been shown to promote digestive health and support immune function. For a dairy-free option, try coconut milk yogurt, which often contains similar probiotic strains.

Kefir, a tangy and effervescent fermented milk drink, is another excellent source of probiotics. Similar to yogurt, it's made by adding live cultures to milk, resulting in a beverage that's rich in beneficial bacteria and easily digestible. Kefir often contains a wider variety of probiotic strains than yogurt, making it a great option for those seeking to diversify their gut microbiome.

Sauerkraut, a traditional fermented cabbage dish, is a surprising but potent source of probiotics. The fermentation process creates an environment that fosters the growth of beneficial bacteria, particularly those from the Lactobacillus family. These bacteria not only contribute to gut health but also add a tangy flavor and crunchy texture to your meals.

Other probiotic-rich foods to consider include kimchi (a spicy Korean fermented cabbage dish), tempeh (a fermented soybean product), and miso (a fermented soybean paste). These foods offer a variety of flavors and textures, making it easy to incorporate probiotics into your daily diet.

While probiotics introduce beneficial bacteria to your gut, prebiotics act as their food source, nourishing and supporting their growth and activity. Think of prebiotics as fertilizer for your gut garden, providing the essential nutrients that your friendly bacteria need to thrive.

Prebiotic-rich foods are typically high in fiber, a type of carbohydrate that our bodies can't digest but that our gut bacteria can ferment. This fermentation process produces short-chain fatty acids, which have numerous health benefits, including improved metabolism, reduced inflammation, and enhanced satiety.

Garlic, onions, and leeks are all excellent sources of prebiotics, thanks to their high content of inulin, a type of soluble fiber that feeds beneficial gut bacteria. These pungent vegetables not only add flavor to your dishes but also support a healthy gut microbiome.

Bananas, another prebiotic powerhouse, contain resistant starch, a type of fiber that resists digestion in the small intestine and reaches the large intestine intact, where it can be fermented by gut bacteria. Resistant starch has been shown to promote the growth of beneficial bacteria, improve insulin sensitivity, and even aid in weight management.

Other prebiotic-rich foods to include in your diet are asparagus, Jerusalem artichokes, dandelion greens, and apples. These foods offer a variety of flavors and textures, making it easy to incorporate prebiotics into your daily meals and snacks.

By strategically combining probiotic and prebiotic foods, you can create a powerful synergy that nurtures your gut microbiome and optimizes your metabolic function. This dynamic duo works together to promote a balanced and diverse gut ecosystem, which in turn supports healthy digestion, immune function, and weight management.

Green Tea and Gut Health: Research on Green Tea's Impact on the Microbiome

The realm of the gut microbiome is an ever-evolving frontier of scientific discovery, teeming with possibilities and implications for our overall health. While the Green Tea Metabolism Makeover has already highlighted the profound connection between gut health and weight management, we're now venturing into the fascinating intersection of green tea and the gut microbiome. Could this ancient beverage hold the key to nurturing a flourishing gut ecosystem, further bolstering our efforts to achieve and maintain a healthy weight?

Emerging research suggests a resounding "yes." While green tea has long been celebrated for its antioxidant and metabolism-boosting properties, its potential impact on the gut microbiome is a relatively new and exciting area of study. Several studies have hinted at green tea's ability to act as a prebiotic, selectively nourishing beneficial gut bacteria and fostering a balanced and thriving microbial community.

Prebiotics, often referred to as "food for probiotics," are non-digestible fibers that stimulate the growth and activity of beneficial bacteria in the gut. These bacteria, in turn, play a crucial role in various bodily functions, including digestion, nutrient absorption, immune function, and even metabolism. By promoting the growth of these friendly microbes, green tea may indirectly contribute to improved gut health, reduced inflammation, and enhanced metabolic function, all of which support our weight loss goals.

The potential prebiotic effects of green tea are attributed to its unique blend of bioactive compounds, particularly catechins. These powerful antioxidants have been shown to selectively inhibit the growth of harmful bacteria while fostering the growth of beneficial bacteria like Bifidobacterium and Lactobacillus. This selective action helps maintain a healthy balance in the gut microbiome, preventing the overgrowth of opportunistic pathogens that can contribute to inflammation and metabolic dysfunction.

Furthermore, green tea's catechins may also influence the gut microbiome by modulating the production of short-chain fatty acids (SCFAs). These beneficial compounds, produced by gut bacteria through the fermentation of dietary fiber, have been linked to numerous health benefits, including improved insulin sensitivity, reduced inflammation, and increased satiety. By promoting the growth of bacteria that produce SCFAs, green tea may indirectly contribute to weight management and metabolic health.

Several studies have shed light on the potential prebiotic effects of green tea. A study published in the Journal of Nutritional Biochemistry found that green tea extract supplementation led to a significant increase in beneficial bacteria and a decrease in harmful bacteria in the gut of obese mice. This shift in gut microbiota composition was associated with improved glucose tolerance and reduced fat accumulation, suggesting that green tea may help combat obesity and metabolic dysfunction by modulating the gut microbiome.

Another study published in the European Journal of Nutrition showed that green tea consumption was associated with a more diverse gut microbiome in humans. Microbial diversity is a key indicator of gut health, as a diverse microbiome is better equipped to perform its various functions and resist colonization by harmful pathogens. By promoting microbial diversity, green tea may help strengthen the gut barrier, reduce inflammation, and support overall health.

While more research is needed to fully understand the complex relationship between green tea and the gut microbiome, these initial findings offer a promising glimpse into the potential of this ancient beverage to support gut health and weight management. By incorporating green tea into your daily routine, you're not only fueling your metabolism and enhancing fat burning but also nurturing the trillions of microbes that call your gut home.

As you embark on your Green Tea Metabolism Makeover journey, embrace the power of green tea as a prebiotic ally, promoting a balanced and thriving gut microbiome. With each cup, you're not just enjoying a delicious and refreshing beverage; you're fostering a healthy gut ecosystem that supports your overall well-being and empowers you to achieve your weight loss goals.

Remember, a healthy gut is a happy gut, and a happy gut is essential for a healthy, vibrant you. So, raise your cup to the power of green tea and let its prebiotic magic work wonders within your gut, paving the way for a transformative journey towards a healthier, leaner, and more energized you.

Chapter 10: Green Tea Beyond Weight Loss: Additional Health Benefits

"Green tea is not just a beverage; it's a journey to a healthier, happier you."

While the transformative power of green tea in the realm of weight loss and metabolism is undeniable, its benefits extend far beyond shedding pounds and boosting energy levels. This ancient elixir, steeped in history and revered across cultures, holds a treasure trove of health-promoting properties that can enhance your overall well-being and protect against chronic diseases.

Imagine green tea as a multi-faceted gem, each facet reflecting a different aspect of its remarkable potential. From its heart-protective antioxidants to its brain-boosting compounds, green tea offers a holistic approach to health that goes beyond the scale.

Let's begin our exploration of green tea's additional health benefits by delving into its impact on cardiovascular health. Heart disease remains the leading cause of death globally, claiming millions of lives each year. However, research suggests that green tea may offer a natural and delicious way to protect your heart and reduce your risk of cardiovascular disease.

Studies have shown that regular consumption of green tea is associated with reduced levels of LDL ("bad") cholesterol and triglycerides, two key risk factors for heart disease. The catechins in green tea, particularly EGCG, have been shown to inhibit the absorption of cholesterol in the gut and promote its excretion from the body. Additionally, green tea may help improve blood vessel function and reduce blood pressure, further protecting your heart and circulatory system.

The benefits of green tea for heart health extend beyond cholesterol and blood pressure reduction. Studies have also suggested that green tea may help prevent blood clots, which can lead to heart attacks and strokes. The antioxidants in green tea may also protect against oxidative stress, a process that damages cells and contributes to the development of atherosclerosis, the buildup of plaque in the arteries.

Beyond its heart-protective effects, green tea also offers a wealth of benefits for brain health. The combination of caffeine and L-theanine in green tea creates a unique synergistic effect that enhances cognitive function, memory, and attention. Caffeine provides a gentle energy boost and increases alertness, while L-theanine promotes relaxation and focus, without the jitters often associated with coffee.

Furthermore, green tea's antioxidant and anti-inflammatory properties may help protect the brain against age-related decline and neurodegenerative diseases like Alzheimer's and Parkinson's. Studies have shown that green tea consumption is associated with a reduced risk of cognitive impairment and dementia, suggesting that this beverage may play a role in preserving brain health throughout our lives.

Green tea's potential benefits extend even further, with emerging research suggesting that it may help protect against certain types of cancer. The antioxidants in green tea, particularly EGCG, have been shown to inhibit the growth of cancer cells and promote their death. While more research is needed to fully understand the mechanisms involved, studies have linked green tea consumption to a reduced risk of several cancers, including breast, colon, prostate, and lung cancer.

In addition to its internal benefits, green tea can also work wonders for your skin. Its antioxidant properties protect the skin from damage caused by free radicals, unstable molecules that can accelerate aging and contribute to wrinkles and fine lines. Green tea also has anti-inflammatory effects, which can help soothe irritated skin and reduce redness. Some studies suggest that green tea may even help protect against skin cancer, although more research is needed in this area.

The versatility of green tea doesn't end there. It's been linked to improved oral health, stronger bones, enhanced immune function, and even a reduced risk of type 2 diabetes. With each cup of green tea you consume, you're not just enjoying a delicious beverage; you're investing in your long-term health and well-being.

As you embark on your Green Tea Metabolism Makeover, remember that the benefits of this ancient elixir extend far beyond weight loss. By incorporating green tea into your daily routine, you're not only fueling your metabolism and supporting your weight loss goals but also nourishing your body from the inside out. You're strengthening your heart, protecting your brain, promoting healthy skin, and reducing your risk of chronic diseases.

The journey toward a healthier you extends beyond simply shedding pounds and boosting metabolism. It encompasses a holistic approach to well-being, fortifying your body against chronic diseases and empowering you to live a long, vibrant life. In the realm of heart health, green tea emerges as a powerful ally, its arsenal of antioxidants and bioactive compounds working tirelessly to protect your cardiovascular system and pave the way for a vibrant and resilient heart.

Imagine your heart as a majestic engine, propelling life-giving blood throughout your body with each rhythmic beat. Its health and vitality are paramount, and green tea, with its remarkable array of benefits, can act as a guardian, shielding your heart from the ravages of time and lifestyle factors.

One of the most significant ways green tea supports heart health is by helping to regulate cholesterol levels. Cholesterol, a waxy substance found in your blood, is essential for building healthy cells and producing hormones. However, too much cholesterol, particularly the "bad" kind known as LDL cholesterol, can build up in your arteries, forming plaques that restrict blood flow and increase the risk of heart attack and stroke. Green tea's catechins, especially the potent EGCG, have been shown to reduce LDL cholesterol levels and triglycerides, another type of fat found in your blood. These compounds work by inhibiting the absorption of cholesterol in the gut and promoting its excretion from the body. They also help prevent the oxidation of LDL cholesterol, a process that makes it more likely to stick to artery walls and form plaque.

Numerous studies have confirmed the cholesterol-lowering effects of green tea. A meta-analysis of 14 randomized controlled trials found that green tea consumption significantly reduced total cholesterol and LDL cholesterol levels, with the most significant reductions seen in those with high cholesterol levels at baseline. Another study published in the American Journal of Clinical Nutrition showed that drinking green tea for 12 weeks led to a significant decrease in LDL cholesterol and triglycerides in adults with high cholesterol.

Beyond its impact on cholesterol, green tea also plays a role in regulating blood pressure, another critical factor in heart health. High blood pressure, also known as hypertension, puts a strain on your heart and blood vessels, increasing the risk of heart attack, stroke, and kidney disease. Studies have shown that regular green tea consumption can lead to modest reductions in both systolic and diastolic blood pressure. The mechanisms behind this effect are not fully understood, but researchers believe that green tea's catechins and other antioxidants may help relax blood vessels and improve their function, leading to lower blood pressure. Additionally, green tea's caffeine content may contribute to a temporary increase in blood pressure, but this effect is typically short-lived and outweighed by the long-term blood pressure-lowering benefits of green tea's other compounds.

In a meta-analysis of nine randomized controlled trials, green tea consumption was associated with a significant reduction in systolic blood pressure, with the most significant effects seen in individuals with hypertension at baseline. Another study published in the Journal of the American College of Nutrition found that drinking green tea for 12 weeks led to a significant decrease in both systolic and diastolic blood pressure in adults with prehypertension or stage 1 hypertension. The cardiovascular benefits of green tea extend beyond cholesterol and blood pressure regulation. Its antioxidant properties play a crucial role in protecting your heart from oxidative stress, a process that damages cells and contributes to the development of atherosclerosis, the buildup of plaque in the arteries. The catechins in green tea, particularly EGCG, neutralize free radicals, unstable molecules that can damage cells and tissues, thus reducing oxidative stress and inflammation.

Furthermore, green tea may also help improve blood vessel function and prevent blood clots, both of which are critical for maintaining a healthy heart and circulatory system. Studies have shown that green tea consumption can increase the production of nitric oxide, a molecule that helps relax blood vessels and improve blood flow. It may also inhibit the activity of platelets, blood cells that play a role in clot formation.

By incorporating green tea into your daily routine, you're not just enjoying a delicious and refreshing beverage; you're also taking proactive steps to protect your heart and reduce your risk of cardiovascular disease. Whether you prefer a steaming cup of sencha, a vibrant matcha latte, or a chilled glass of green tea-infused water, each sip is a gift to your cardiovascular system.

As you embark on your Green Tea Metabolism Makeover journey, remember that a healthy heart is the foundation of a healthy life. By nourishing your body with wholesome foods, engaging in regular exercise, and embracing the power of green tea, you're creating a lifestyle that promotes not only weight loss but also long-term cardiovascular health and vitality.

Green Tea and Brain Health: Boosting Cognitive Function and Protecting Against Neurodegenerative Diseases

In the quest for a healthier, more vibrant life, we often focus on the physical aspects of well-being: shedding pounds, toning muscles, and boosting energy levels. But true wellness encompasses more than just a fit physique; it includes a sharp and agile mind, capable of learning, adapting, and thriving in an ever-changing world. As we delve deeper into the transformative power of green tea, we uncover its remarkable potential to nourish not only our bodies but also our brains. This ancient elixir, with its unique blend of compounds, holds the key to unlocking a world of cognitive enhancement, memory preservation, and protection against neurodegenerative diseases.

Imagine your brain as a vast and intricate network of neurons, constantly firing signals and forging connections that shape your thoughts, emotions, and memories. Green tea, with its combination of caffeine and L-theanine, acts as a gentle stimulant and a calming agent, creating a harmonious balance that enhances cognitive function and promotes mental clarity. Caffeine, the well-known stimulant found in coffee and tea, works by blocking adenosine receptors in the brain, a neurotransmitter that promotes sleepiness and relaxation. By inhibiting adenosine, caffeine increases alertness, focus, and reaction time. However, caffeine alone can also lead to jitters, anxiety, and a subsequent crash. This is where L-theanine, the unique amino acid found in green tea, comes into play.

L-theanine counteracts the stimulating effects of caffeine, promoting a state of calm alertness that is both relaxed and focused. It works by increasing the levels of GABA, a neurotransmitter that inhibits overstimulation in the brain, and dopamine, a neurotransmitter associated with pleasure and reward. L-theanine also modulates the levels of serotonin, a neurotransmitter that plays a key role in regulating mood, sleep, and appetite. The synergistic combination of caffeine and L-theanine in green tea creates a unique cognitive boost that is both energizing and calming. Studies have shown that this combination can improve attention, reaction time, and accuracy on cognitive tasks, making it a valuable tool for students, professionals, and anyone seeking to optimize their mental performance.

But the benefits of green tea for brain health extend far beyond cognitive enhancement. Research suggests that its potent antioxidants, particularly EGCG, may have neuroprotective effects, potentially reducing the risk of neurodegenerative diseases like Alzheimer's and Parkinson's.

Alzheimer's disease, the most common form of dementia, is characterized by a progressive decline in cognitive function, memory loss, and behavioral changes. While the exact cause of Alzheimer's remains unknown, it's believed to be associated with the buildup of amyloid plaques and tau tangles in the brain, which disrupt communication between neurons and lead to cell death.

Studies have shown that EGCG can inhibit the formation of amyloid plaques and tau tangles, suggesting that green tea may help protect against the development of Alzheimer's disease. Additionally, green tea's anti-inflammatory properties may help reduce neuroinflammation, a key contributor to the progression of Alzheimer's and other neurodegenerative diseases.

Parkinson's disease, another common neurodegenerative disorder, is characterized by tremors, stiffness, and difficulty with movement and coordination. It's caused by the loss of dopamine-producing neurons in the brain, which are essential for controlling movement. While there's no cure for Parkinson's disease, studies suggest that green tea may help slow its progression and alleviate some of its symptoms.

EGCG has been shown to protect dopamine-producing neurons from damage and may even promote their regeneration. Additionally, green tea's anti-inflammatory properties may help reduce neuroinflammation associated with Parkinson's disease.

The potential neuroprotective effects of green tea are not limited to Alzheimer's and Parkinson's diseases. Studies have also suggested that green tea may help protect against other neurodegenerative disorders, such as Huntington's disease and amyotrophic lateral sclerosis (ALS). While more research is needed to fully understand the mechanisms involved, these findings suggest that green tea may be a valuable tool for preserving brain health and reducing the risk of cognitive decline.

In addition to its protective effects, green tea may also help improve cognitive function and memory in individuals already experiencing age-related decline or mild cognitive impairment. Studies have shown that green tea consumption can improve attention, working memory, and overall cognitive performance in older adults. These benefits may be attributed to green tea's ability to enhance blood flow to the brain, protect against oxidative stress, and modulate neurotransmitter levels.

As you embark on your Green Tea Metabolism Makeover journey, consider the profound impact that this ancient beverage can have on your brain health. By incorporating green tea into your daily routine, you're not just supporting your weight loss goals but also nourishing your mind and promoting cognitive vitality. Whether you're a student, a professional, or simply someone who values a sharp and agile mind, green tea can be a valuable ally in your quest for optimal brain health.

Remember, the benefits of green tea extend far beyond the physical realm. It's a holistic elixir that nourishes both your body and your mind, empowering you to live a healthier, happier, and more fulfilling life.

Green Tea and Skin Health: Promoting a Radiant Complexion

While the Green Tea Metabolism Makeover journey focuses on igniting your inner fire and transforming your body from within, the radiance of good health often shines through on the outside as well. Your skin, the largest organ of your body, is a reflection of your overall well-being. And as you embark on this transformative path, green tea emerges as a powerful ally, not only for your metabolism but also for the health and beauty of your skin.

Imagine your skin as a delicate canvas, exposed to the elements and the ravages of time. Free radicals, unstable molecules generated by environmental pollutants, UV radiation, and even our own metabolic processes, can wreak havoc on this canvas, causing damage that manifests as wrinkles, fine lines, age spots, and a dull complexion. But fear not, for green tea, with its potent antioxidant arsenal, acts as a protective shield, neutralizing these free radicals and safeguarding your skin's youthful glow.

At the heart of green tea's skin-protective properties are its catechins, particularly EGCG. These antioxidants scavenge free radicals, preventing them from damaging collagen and elastin, the proteins that give our skin its structure and elasticity. By neutralizing free radicals, green tea helps maintain the integrity of your skin's connective tissues, reducing the appearance of wrinkles and fine lines and promoting a smoother, more youthful complexion. But green tea's benefits for skin health go beyond just antioxidant protection. It also possesses anti-inflammatory properties that can help soothe irritated skin and reduce redness. This is particularly beneficial for individuals with conditions like acne and eczema, where inflammation plays a significant role.

Studies have shown that applying green tea extract topically can reduce sebum production, the oily substance that can clog pores and contribute to acne breakouts. It also has antibacterial properties that can help combat the bacteria associated with acne. For individuals with eczema, green tea's anti-inflammatory effects can help soothe itchy and irritated skin, providing much-needed relief.

Furthermore, green tea may help stimulate collagen production, the protein that gives our skin its structure and firmness. As we age, collagen production naturally declines, leading to sagging skin and wrinkles. By promoting collagen synthesis, green tea can help maintain your skin's elasticity and youthful appearance.

The benefits of green tea for skin health are not just theoretical; numerous studies have confirmed its efficacy in improving various skin conditions. A study published in the Journal of the American Academy of Dermatology found that applying a green tea extract cream to the skin significantly reduced sun damage and improved skin elasticity. Another study in the Journal of Investigative Dermatology showed that green tea extract reduced sebum production and improved acne lesions in individuals with mild to moderate acne.

In addition to topical applications, consuming green tea can also benefit your skin from the inside out. The antioxidants in green tea help protect your skin cells from damage caused by free radicals, UV radiation, and other environmental stressors. They also support the production of collagen and elastin, promoting a healthy and radiant complexion. As part of your Green Tea Metabolism Makeover, incorporating green tea into your skincare routine can be a simple yet effective way to enhance your skin's health and beauty. Consider using green tea-infused cleansers, toners, moisturizers, and masks to reap the benefits of its antioxidant and anti-inflammatory properties. You can also try brewing a strong cup of green tea and using it as a facial toner or mist. The tannins in green tea can help tighten pores and reduce oiliness, while the antioxidants provide a protective shield against environmental damage.

Remember, healthy skin is a reflection of a healthy body. By nourishing your body with a balanced diet, regular exercise, adequate sleep, and stress management techniques, you're creating the ideal environment for your skin to thrive. And by incorporating green tea into your daily routine, you're providing your skin with an extra layer of protection and nourishment, helping you achieve a radiant complexion that glows from within.

As you continue your journey towards a healthier, more vibrant you, remember that beauty is not just skin deep. It's a reflection of your overall well-being, a radiant glow that emanates from a body and mind in harmony. Embrace the power of green tea, both internally and externally, and let its transformative properties guide you towards a healthier, happier, and more radiant you.

CONCLUSION

Congratulations! You've journeyed through the transformative pages of "The Green Tea Metabolism Makeover," and in doing so, you've unlocked the secrets to harnessing the power of green tea for a healthier, leaner, and more vibrant you. As we close this chapter of your journey, let's reflect on the profound impact this ancient elixir can have on your life and empower you to continue your path toward lasting wellness.

Throughout this book, we've explored the multifaceted nature of green tea, its rich history intertwined with its remarkable scientific validation. We've delved into the intricate workings of your metabolism, understanding how green tea's unique compounds, particularly the mighty EGCG, can ignite your fat-burning potential and enhance your body's ability to utilize energy efficiently.
We've embarked on a culinary adventure, discovering the delightful ways in which green tea can be woven into your daily meals and snacks. From energizing matcha lattes to refreshing green tea smoothies and guilt-free desserts, we've learned to savor the flavors of this ancient beverage while nourishing our bodies from the inside out. The Green Tea Metabolism Food Pyramid has served as our compass, guiding us towards balanced meals that support our weight loss goals and overall health.

We've also embraced the power of movement, recognizing that exercise is not just about shedding pounds but also about strengthening our hearts, building resilient muscles, and fortifying our bones. The Green Tea Workout Plan has provided a roadmap for incorporating both cardio and strength training into our routines, maximizing fat burning and promoting overall fitness.
But the Green Tea Metabolism Makeover is not just about diet and exercise; it's about cultivating a holistic approach to health that encompasses the mind, body, and spirit. We've explored the profound connection between stress and weight gain, learning to manage stress through mindful practices and harnessing the calming power of L-theanine in green tea.

We've also delved into the crucial role of sleep in weight management, understanding how quality sleep supports hormonal balance, metabolism, and overall well-being. By prioritizing sleep and incorporating green tea into our bedtime routines, we've created a sanctuary for rest and rejuvenation.

Beyond weight loss, we've uncovered the myriad of additional health benefits that green tea offers. From protecting our hearts and brains to promoting healthy skin and reducing the risk of chronic diseases, green tea is truly an elixir for longevity and vitality. We've even explored the emerging research on green tea's potential prebiotic effects, suggesting that it may play a role in nurturing a healthy gut microbiome, further supporting our overall health and metabolic function.

As you reflect on your journey through these pages, remember that the Green Tea Metabolism Makeover is not a quick fix or a fad diet. It's a lifestyle transformation, a commitment to nourishing your body and mind with wholesome foods, mindful practices, and the invigorating power of green tea. It's about embracing a sustainable approach to health that empowers you to achieve your weight loss goals while cultivating a deeper connection with your body and the world around you.

The 28-day plan outlined in this book is just the beginning. It's a springboard to a lifetime of healthy habits and mindful choices. As you continue your journey, remember the key principles we've explored:

- **Embrace the power of green tea:** Make it a daily ritual, savoring its flavors and reaping its numerous health benefits.
- **Nourish your body with whole foods:** Prioritize vegetables, fruits, whole grains, lean proteins, and healthy fats, building your plate for success with the Green Tea Metabolism Food Pyramid as your guide.
- **Move your body with joy:** Find activities you love and incorporate them into your routine, whether it's dancing, swimming, hiking, or strength training.
- **Manage stress and prioritize sleep:** Cultivate mindfulness, practice relaxation techniques, and create a sleep sanctuary to support your overall well-being.
- **Celebrate your progress:** Acknowledge your achievements, no matter how small, and reward yourself for your hard work and dedication.

As you continue on this path, remember that setbacks are a natural part of any journey. Don't be discouraged if you encounter challenges or slip-ups along the way. Instead, view them as opportunities for growth and learning. Embrace the process, be kind to yourself, and celebrate every step forward.

Green Tea Enthusiasts, Your Voice Matters!

Hey there, wellness warrior in the making!

I hope "The Green Tea Metabolism Makeover" has ignited your passion for a healthier lifestyle and fueled your journey towards a more vibrant you.

Now, I'm turning to you, the heart of the green tea community. Your experiences, insights, and triumphs on this 28-day journey are incredibly valuable. By sharing your honest thoughts in a review on Amazon, you're not only helping other health-conscious individuals discover the transformative power of green tea, but you're also shaping the future of holistic wellness.
Your feedback fuels my creativity and inspires me to continue crafting resources that empower you to become the best version of yourself. Whether you've mastered a new green tea recipe, conquered a challenging workout, or simply found inner peace through mindful eating, your review makes a difference.

How to Share Your 5-Star Transformation Story on Amazon:

5. Visit the Amazon page for "The Green Tea Metabolism Makeover."
6. Scroll down to the "Customer Reviews" section.
7. Click on the "Write a customer review" button.
8. Give the book a well-deserved 5-star rating and share your inspiring transformation story!

It's that simple! Your voice matters, and together, we can make the green tea community even stronger and more vibrant.

Thank you for being a part of this transformative adventure!

Evelyn Green (Author of "The Green Tea Metabolism Makeover")